What people are saying about the power of *Ten Years Thinner*

"I lost 33 pounds in six weeks without feeling hungry. I'm living proof that this program works."

— GREG, 34

"My friends on Weight Watchers are afraid to eat. Every pound they lose seems to be a struggle. One lady told me she's always starving, but she's afraid to eat because she knows she'll just regain all the weight she's lost. They can't believe the results I've gotten on *Ten Years Thinner* eating as much as I do. I am NEVER hungry, but I'm still losing pounds and inches."

— DARLENE, 43

"The *Ten Years Thinner* program delivers amazing results in such a short time. I would totally recommend it to anyone, whether they are newly embarking on a healthy lifestyle or just wanting to improve their current level of fitness."

— KIM, 39

"I lost ten pounds in four weeks on the *Ten Years Thinner* program. After the first two days, I didn't have any more cravings. By the end of the first week, my energy was increasing and I already felt stronger. By the end of the second week, my clothes were fitting differently and my arms were noticeably more toned. Within a month, I'd lost five inches off my waist. But the best part was my butt. By the end of the six weeks, I actually had one!"

— LISA, 36

"I was motivated to try *Ten Years Thinner* after learning I had high cholesterol. I followed the program for six weeks and, without medication, my cholesterol levels fell to well within the normal range."

— DEANNE, 35

"I lost 12 pounds in three weeks without craving junk food or feeling hungry between meals."

— ALEX, 35

"I lost pounds and inches in the first week. My energy soared during the second week. By the third week, my clothes were fitting very differently. I would definitely recommend this program to my friends. I think if they were to try it for three weeks and see the results, they'd be hooked."

— COLLEEN, 43

"I recently underwent two major surgeries and was laid up for about three months. After my first week doing the *Ten Years Thinner* exercise program, I could already see and feel my body getting stronger by the day. After six weeks, my body was even leaner than before my surgery."

— HEATHER, 38

"My biggest concern when I started the *Ten Years Thinner* program was that I wouldn't be able to give up the bad carbs. I love pasta; I love bread; I love french fries. But my cravings were completely eliminated within the first few days. *Gone.* And I don't miss those foods. The program literally changed what I have an appetite for. And I got amazing results! I dropped six pounds in the first week, and I lost 21 pounds in under two months. I've now lost a total of 28 pounds and am in better shape than I was in my early twenties."

— MATT, 38

"I saw amazing improvements in just six weeks! This program changed my life; it made me realize that eating right and exercising don't have to be a chore."

— FRANCOISE, 26

"Between raising a toddler, working a full-time job, and running a small business, it's a challenge for me to find time to exercise. The *Ten Years Thinner* workout fits my life because it only takes 25 minutes a day and I don't have to leave my living room to do it."

— MELISSA, 36

"When I hear the term diet, I think restriction. But this program isn't restrictive. I'm never hungry. Sometimes I actually have trouble finishing the portions. I also never have cravings. In fact, on the cheat days, I usually forget to cheat!"

— CATHY, 31

"The diet is very easy to follow and extremely versatile. If anything, it's streamlined my eating."

— LAURIE, 43

"The *Ten Years Thinner* program never left me with uncontrollable cravings like Atkins did. This program works because it puts you on the road to results and gives you the tools you need to stay there."

— DON, 32

"I am a police officer and have always strived to have a high level of fitness. The *Ten Years Thinner* program allowed me to lose fat, gain muscle, increase my energy, and end food cravings. I finally got rid of the spare tire that had been stubbornly resisting my efforts for years."

— CHRISTOPHER, 35

"I have two kids under the age of six, a full-time job, and a husband who works ten- to twelve-hour days, six days a week. I've tried many times to fit regular exercise into my schedule. *Ten Years Thinner* is so simple and so convenient, it's the first program I've ever found that both fits into my life and produces results. I have a pair of pants that I haven't been able to wear since 1996. Today, they fit me better than they did when I bought them in 1992. Maybe the book should have been called Fifteen Years Thinner!"

— JILLIAN, 38

TEN YEARS THINNER

TEN YEARS THINNER

,,,,,

6 WEEKS TO A LEANER, YOUNGER-LOOKING YOU!

CHRISTINE LYDON, M.D.

Da Capo

LIFE
LONG

A Member of the Perseus Books Group

Copyright 2008 Christine Lydon
Photographs © Mark Richards Studios

Designed by Trish Wilkinson
Set in 11-point Adobe Caslon

Library of Congress Cataloging-in-Publication Data

Lydon, Christine, 1966-
    Ten years thinner : 6 weeks to a leaner, younger-looking you! / Christine Lydon. — 1st ed.
        p.   cm.
    Includes bibliographical references.
    ISBN-13: 978-0-7382-1102-2 (hardcover : alk. paper)
    ISBN-10: 0-7382-1102-8 (hardcover : alk. paper) 1. Weight loss. 2. Physical fitness.
I. Title.
RM222.2.L93 2007
613.2'5—dc22   2007035609

First Da Capo Press edition 2008

Published by Da Capo Press
A Member of the Perseus Books Group
www.dacapopress.com

Note: The information in this book is true and complete to the best of our knowledge. This book is intended only as an informative guide for those wishing to know more about health issues. In no way is this book intended to replace, countermand, or conflict with the advice given to you by your own physician. The ultimate decision concerning care should be made between you and your doctor. We strongly recommend you follow his or her advice. Information in this book is general and is offered with no guarantees on the part of the author or Da Capo Press. The author and publisher disclaim all liability in connection with the use of this book. The names and identifying details of people associated with events described in this book have been changed. Any similarity to actual persons is coincidental.

Da Capo Press books are available at special discounts for bulk purchases in the U.S. by corporations, institutions, and other organizations. For more information, please contact the Special Markets Department at the Perseus Books Group, 2300 Chestnut Street, Suite 200, Philadelphia, PA 19103, or call (800) 255-1514, or e-mail special.markets@perseusbooks.com.

10 9 8 7 6 5 4 3 2 1

This book is dedicated to everyone who has ever starved themselves, or skipped meals, or compulsively counted calories in a feckless effort to shed pounds that always came back.

This book is dedicated to everyone who has ever endured the guilt of having spent a small fortune on a gym membership they never used, or workout videos they never watched, or exercise equipment that now sits collecting dust in their garage.

This book is dedicated to everyone who has ever gazed into their bathroom mirror and disparaged their reflection, wishing they could turn back the clock and look and feel the way they did ten years ago.

Contents

Acknowledgments

Once upon a time, on the tiny island of Recovered Dreams, there lived a voracious wizard. Although fabulously wealthy, the wizard possessed only the basest of magical powers, having amassed his fortune pedaling transient glamours—spells of illusory pulchritude that wore off after a few hours. One day, the wizard heard rumors of a woman who dwelled within the craggy ridges of a faraway land, a sorceress who'd discovered the secret to everlasting youth and beauty. The wizard realized that such powerful magic could make him as rich as a king, so he summoned her to his gem-encrusted palace, and in exchange for the secret to everlasting youth and beauty, he offered the sorceress riches beyond her wildest dreams. Seduced by the notion of a gem-encrusted palace of her own, the sorceress acquiesced and whispered her secret into the wizard's ear. But as he listened, a cruel smile curled his vermillion lips. "How simple!" he thought to himself. "Hardly a secret worth the riches I've promised."

I can never adequately express the appreciation I feel for the team of white knights who rescued me from the wizard's dungeon: David Rudich, Matthew Saver, Micheal Gross of the Author's Guild, Jonathan Wolfert, and my amazing agent, Rick Broadhead, without whose sympathetic support, encouragement, and wise counsel, the *Ten Years Thinner* program never would have existed, and its frazzled creator would now be languishing in obscurity. I also want to thank all the friends and family (especially Heather Wunder, Christine Kenny, Jill Davies, Gabe Pryce-Jones, Sabrina Mance, Kris Cooper, my brother, Jeff, and my sisters, Marcy and Miriam) who stood by me through those dark times and who, despite suffering countless earfuls of woe, never once informed me what a tedious bore I had become.

But I owe my biggest debt of gratitude to the dozens of volunteers who, in addition to trusting me with their health and well-being, diligently completed questionnaires and compliance forms, endured the indignity of tape measures and weigh-ins, and bravely donned their most revealing undergarments so I could track their progress with awkward snapshots. The results you achieved surpassed my wildest expectations, and your impressions and feedback were instrumental in making this the most effective weight loss program in existence! Special thanks to: Russel Mack and Pemberton Fire Rescue for allowing me to periodically turn the engine bay into a fitness studio; Shantelle Clarke, Todd McGivern, Clau Boudrias, Meghan Menzel, Caprii Mohammed, and Greg and Ingrid Burt for sailing uncharted seas; and Darlene Knapton, Matt Davies, Jillian Edwards, Colleen Alfier, Deanne Downey, Laurie Fairbanks, Kim Saulnier, Melissa Kish, Chris Raabis, Lisa Storoshenko, and Dorothy Swanson for providing such impassioned testimonials, for donating so many delicious recipes, and for helping me elevate my own culinary contributions from edible to delectable. (I never claimed to be a cook.)

And last, but certainly not least, I would like to express my heartfelt appreciation to my sage and gentle handlers, Marnie Cochran of Da Capo Press and Andrea Magyar of Penguin Group (Canada). Thank you both, a million times over, for *everything*!

The Blueprint

————— 🥚🥚🥚🥚🥚 —————

"I've never felt better. I realize now that, for many years,
I was sticking my head in the sand about
what I was putting in my body." — MATT, 38

"I felt changes right away. My sleep, my digestion, and my energy
levels all improved within the first few days. I felt calmer, stronger,
and fitter by the end of the first week. How you feel on this
program really keeps you motivated to continue!" — JILLIAN, 38

"The *Ten Years Thinner* program changed my life. My confidence
has increased and I feel wonderful." — LISA, 35

————— 🥚🥚🥚🥚🥚 —————

Introduction

Although the fruits that bore *Ten Years Thinner* began to ripen within the venerable corridors of the Yale University School of Medicine, the seeds of my revolutionary weight loss program actually germinated many years later beneath the leaky roof of the local fire hall.

At the time, I was a volunteer firefighter with Pemberton Fire Rescue and my crew was in the process of gearing down after a house fire. We were all standing in our underwear when the only other female member of our 30-man department, a devoted, 23-year-old gym-goer named Cheryl who earned her living as a utilities technician, turned to me and said, "No matter how many hours I spend on that damn treadmill, I still can't get rid of these ugly saddlebags. And no matter how many crunches I do, I still have this layer of flab on my tummy. Your thighs and butt are so toned—and your stomach is always flat. I just don't get it. Aren't you, like, forty years old? *How do you do it?!*"

I told Cheryl that I was in the process of developing a diet and exercise program that I believed would promote fat loss faster than if she were to continue spending all her spare time on a human hamster wheel. I warned her that if she wanted to try it, she would have to give up her cardio addiction—no more treadmill or StairMaster or Lifecycle—or she would short-circuit the physiological mechanisms that my program was intended to harness. Faced with the delicious prospect of *never* having to do another boring cardio workout *ever again*, Cheryl leaped at the opportunity. So, I grabbed a clipboard from Engine 13 and, on the back of a blank rig-check form, I jotted down a brief, simple-to-follow exercise routine. I told Cheryl that the entire workout probably wouldn't take her more than 20 minutes to do and recommended that she do it religiously, five or six days per week. I also made a list of ten dietary guidelines that conformed to my nutritional theories.

Six days later, Cheryl and I were again gathered in the fire hall gearing down after attending an emergency involving an overturned propane truck. Cheryl slid her suspenders off her shoulders and, as her trousers dropped around her ankles, she stepped out of her bunker gear and proudly announced, "I can already see a difference!"

But perhaps I am getting ahead of my story. . . .

When friends, family members, or business associates have physique dilemmas, nutritional concerns, or questions relating to general good health, they come to me. I earned my MD from Yale in 1994, but unlike most of my peers, I chose not to practice medicine in the traditional sense. While most MD's earn their living treating disease, I vowed I would earn mine by preventing it.

After forgoing a surgical career, I went on to build a flourishing fitness practice with a client list that boasted music producers, supermodels, and Academy Award–winners in Los Angeles. I was one of very few nutritionists or trainers who could honestly say that my techniques were consistent with cutting edge scientific theories. But that's not the main reason I was attracting an A-list clientele: On top of my Ivy League pedigree and research background, *I walked the walk!* I was a recognizable physique model making regular appearances in all the major health magazines. People placed their trust in my methods because I was a living, breathing example of how proper nutrition and training could sculpt a physique.

Plus, my clients got great results!

Rather than go to a health club, most of my celebrity patrons preferred to save time and avoid interruptions by working out in their home exercise facilities. At the height of my private consulting practice, I was spending six days a week scrambling from Beverly Hills to Malibu to the Hollywood Hills and back again, putting in the same long hours I'd left a career in surgery to avoid in the first place.

Ironically, as my training business grew, I found I had less and less time to devote to my own athletic endeavors. I stopped going to my karate class. I quit my roller hockey team. I stored my surfboard in the garage next to my mountain bike where they both sat collecting dust. And I started to rely more and more heavily on the cardio theater at my health club to meet my exercise needs. My gym was conveniently located within walking distance of my apartment and it was open past midnight. After an exhausting 12 hour day, I'd wander in there late at night and climb aboard a Lifecycle, or a treadmill, or if the mood struck me, maybe a StairMaster. Then I'd spin or jog or step within my so-called "fat-burning zone" for 45 minutes to an hour. But despite all the time I devoted to pedaling and running and climbing in place, for the first time in my entire life, an insidious layer of flab was slowly claiming my hips and thighs.

I distinctly remember modeling for a photo shoot for *Muscle and Fitness Magazine*. The photographer, with whom I'd worked on numerous occasions, took me aside and told me in no uncertain terms that I wasn't in my usual shape. He commented that over the past year, my physique had become subtly flabbier, and that my lower body was slowly losing definition. He warned me that if I didn't lean out, the magazines would have no further use for me. I knew if I let my physique slide, it would not only impact my reputation as a personal trainer, it would mean the end of my career as a fitness model and spokesperson.

I panicked.

I doubled the time I spent at the gym every night, devoting up to two hours a session to the various human hamster wheels. But the extra effort didn't make a bit of difference! In fact, it seemed like the more time I spent doing cardio, the softer I got.

I started to take a good, hard look at the path my life was taking. Ostensibly, I'd left a promising career in surgery to educate people about healthy living, but the only individuals now benefiting from my expertise were a handful of wealthy celebrities. It frustrated me to realize that my career path had diverged so widely from my noble aspirations.

I decided to take an extended hiatus from my celebrity training business and get as far away from the rat race as possible. An interest in snowboarding drew me to Whistler, British Columbia, where, for the first time in my entire adult life, I didn't join a health club. Getting out of the gym and away from the treadmill had a tremendous impact on my physique. After just a few weeks of snowboarding, my legs and thighs were leaner and more toned than ever before—despite the fact that *the total amount of time I actually spent exercising had decreased by more than half!* Not to mention the fact that none of the exercise I was getting called for lengthy aerobic sessions.

My puzzling physical transformation flew in the face of everything I held to be true about exercise and weight loss. I began to question whether or not the total number of calories burned during a given activity was really an accurate predictor of weight loss. I wondered if some activities were more likely to stimulate fat burning regardless of the immediate energy expenditure. In other words, could certain forms of exercise be used to program the body so that it became more efficient at fat burning?

That's when my fellow firefighter, Cheryl the cardio queen, gave me a golden opportunity to test my hypothesis. Like many of the individuals I have counseled over the years, Cheryl was disappointed that, despite all the time she devoted to cardiovascular activity, she was unable to achieve the firm, toned physique that someone nearly twice her age made look easy. But after just six days following my diet and exercise recommendations, Cheryl was already noticeably leaner. She wasn't shy about giving me credit for her new look, and pretty soon all the firemen's girlfriends and wives wanted to try my "miracle" program.

I decided to take advantage of the sudden interest and recruit volunteers for an informal clinical trial. Although I deliberately limited the group to 15 previously inactive women with relatively sedentary professions, every one of my test subjects, without exception, experienced significant results. Perhaps even more remarkable, like Cheryl, they all started to see changes *within the first week*! By the end of the six-week trial period, almost everyone had to buy new pants.

The overwhelming success of my first clinical study spawned a series of informal trials. To date, the *Ten Years Thinner* program has helped individuals of all ages and fitness backgrounds shed hundreds of pounds of unwanted fat. In six weeks or less, my program firms hips and thighs, elevates rear ends, defines shoulders and arms, flattens tummies, diminishes the appearance of cellulite, boosts energy levels, and may help reduce symptoms of Irritable Bowel Syndrome, acne, asthma, and migraine headaches. Moreover, even two and three years later, graduates of the *Ten Years Thinner* trials have, by and large, maintained not just their weight loss, but their healthy eating habits and active lifestyles.

WHAT TO EXPECT

Chapters 1 through 7 of *Ten Years Thinner* explore the pivotal roles that nutrition and physical activity play in shaping your healthy body. These chapters provide a coherent framework for the six-week diet and exercise program, explained in detail in Chapters 8 and 9. Chapter 10 addresses the challenge of making the essential principles of the *Ten Years Thinner* program a permanent part of your long, lean, healthy life.

The *Ten Years Thinner* meal plan, which emphasizes healthy protein, carbohydrate, and fat sources, calls for the gradual elimination and reintroduction of specific foods. This organization permits an objective self-evaluation, providing you the opportunity to identify particular foods to which you may be sensitive so you can reduce or avoid their consumption in the future. Rest assured, the dietary recommendations *do not* involve calorie counting, complicated point systems, or messy portion measuring. Best of all, there are no upper limits on healthy choice food consumption, so you never feel hungry or deprived.

The *Ten Years Thinner* exercise program demands only a 20- to 25-minute daily time commitment and a very minimal level of initial fitness. Because the workouts do not require any complicated exercise equipment or even a dedicated workout space, they can be done virtually anywhere, anytime, and by anyone. Between their simplicity and brevity, even the busiest working mother was able to fit the *Ten Years Thinner* exercise routines into her hectic schedule and enjoy fast, tangible results.

The program itself is divided into two phases, each of three weeks' duration. Regardless of your prior fitness level, you will begin to notice subtle changes in your physique within the first week or two. By the completion of Phase 1, your hips, thighs, and tummy will feel firmer. Your arms and back will show increased definition. Cellulite will seem less conspicuous. Love handles and saddlebags will begin to contract and tighten. In addition, you will feel stronger and more coordinated. Your energy levels will be improved, engendering new self-confidence and an elevated mood. You will be looking forward to the upcoming challenges of Phase 2!

For many, Phase 2 is the most dynamic and exciting part of their journey. Many graduates of the *Ten Years Thinner* program found that their fat loss seemed to accelerate between weeks three and four and they shed the greatest number of cumulative inches from their waist, arms, back, thighs, and hips between days 22 and 42. Your body will literally metamorphose before your eyes as every passing week brings visible, tangible changes.

RESIST THE TEMPTATION
TO SKIP AHEAD!

I know you bought this book because you want to look and feel ten years younger, firmer, and more energized. And I bet you are so eager to begin your journey to physique firming, fat burning, metabolic overdrive that you might be tempted to skip ahead a few chapters to get to the meal plan and exercise program.

Patience, dear reader!

Unlike most other diet books, programs, pills, and weight loss contraptions, *Ten Years Thinner* is not a magic bullet. Granted, even if you were to approach the *Ten Years Thinner* program with a quick-fix attitude, you would probably see the dramatic results you expected during the first six weeks. However, without a fundamental understanding of how and why this program works, it would be difficult, if not impossible, for you to establish the eating and exercise habits that would guarantee your firm physique lasts a lifetime.

By our very nature, humans like to push the envelope. We like to see what we can get away with. We feel better if we have a sense of control, especially where our bodies are concerned. I do not want to simply tell you what to do. At every step, I believe it is very important to your long-term success that you understand *why* you are doing what you are doing. Don't get me wrong: Following the *Ten Years Thinner* program will not be unpleasant, time consuming, or complicated. Nevertheless, no matter how simple and enjoyable the process might be, breaking old habits presents a challenge for everyone. Experience has taught me that people are infinitely more likely to adhere to a prescribed eating plan or exercise program if they have a basic understanding of how and why the routine works.

It will only require a small amount of your time to read the upcoming chapters, but the knowledge you gain will help guarantee that your soon-to-be firm physique lasts a lifetime. So please, resist the temptation to skip ahead; read this book as it was meant to be read.

Although none of this is rocket science, for the sake of completeness, there are times that I touch on some rather involved scientific concepts. Be aware that this information is not intended to confuse or frustrate, nor were the following pages written to be memorized. At the end of each chapter or subchapter you will find a brief review of key points distilled from the preceding paragraphs for the purpose of highlighting and reinforcing important ideas. For example:

THE LEAN ESSENTIALS:

- You will increase your chances of long-term success if you read each chapter, in order, and resist the temptation to skip ahead.

- You will not need to memorize the contents of this book. For easy reference, a summary of key points is included at the end of each chapter or subchapter.

- Smile. A thinner, younger, healthier-looking you is just weeks away!

———— ❧❧❧❧❧ ————

"I've tried every diet you can think of from cabbage soup to Weight Watchers. Nothing has given me faster results than the *Ten Years Thinner* program." — LISA, 35

"This is the first diet I've ever gone on where I haven't felt famished and exhausted." — DARLENE, 43

"*Ten Years Thinner* works because it is precisely what other programs are not. If you're looking for another diet gimmick, you've come to the wrong place." — DON, 32

"I highly recommend this excellent program for its fabulous results and how conveniently it fits into your schedule!" — HEATHER, 38

"The program was a lot easier than I thought it was going to be, and the longer I was on it, the easier it got." — JILLIAN, 38

"The fundamental reason this program worked for me was because it wasn't about *restricting* behavior, it was about *changing* it." — MATT, 38

"I would recommend *Ten Years Thinner* to anyone serious about their health." — MELISSA, 36

———— ❧❧❧❧❧ ————

CHAPTER 1

The Un-Diet

What would you say if I told you that you could have a dramatically improved physique in just six weeks? What if I could guarantee that, 42 days from today, you will barely recognize your own reflection? Staring back from the depths of your bathroom mirror, picture someone with slimmer hips, firmer thighs, tighter buns, flatter abs, more defined arms, and clearer, younger-looking skin. And that familiar stranger will be smiling—and not just because you look great; you also *feel* great. Your energy will be higher than it's been in years; your mood will be positive; you will be well rested and know you can handle whatever your busy life throws your way.

Heard it all before? Does it sound a little too good to be true? Do you have the uneasy feeling that deprivation, suffering, and cravings are lurking just around the corner? Maybe with some complicated calculations and impossibly involved recipes thrown in for good measure? If you aren't a little skeptical, you really should be. The vast majority of today's diet books, weight loss products, and exercise gadgets are nothing more than faddy gimmicks that contradict the basic machinery of human physiology and, as a result, are doomed to fail.

Well, *Ten Years Thinner* isn't like other diet books. Rather than *defy* natural laws, the *Ten Years Thinner* program harnesses them. This program is not a fad or a quick fix. It doesn't call for the radical elimination of entire food groups or hours of tedious calisthenics. What you are holding in your hands is a simple, sustainable road map to the physique you've always dreamed of having, a program that will give you rapid, dramatic results that you will begin to see and feel within the first week.

How can I be so sure that this program will work for you?

Because this book is not just about weight loss. This book is about regaining physiological stability so that your body performs like the finely tuned, fat-burning machine it was designed to be. Unlike other weight loss plans, the *Ten Years Thinner* program will not turn you into a smaller, flabbier, hungrier version of your former self. It will not leave you exhausted, depleted, and primed for re-newed weight gain. On the contrary, this program will melt unwanted fat while it tones your muscles, leaving you sated, energetic, and lean.

To make the dietary transition to stable physiology and a balanced equilib-rium as easy as possible, this book includes a detailed meal plan, extensive food lists, and dozens of quick, easy recipes that take all of the guesswork out of eat-ing for a firm, younger-looking physique. The meal plan, which emphasizes healthy protein, carbohydrate, and fat sources, involves no calorie counting, no complicated "point systems," and no messy portion measuring. There are no up-per limits placed on healthy choice food consumption, so you never have to feel hungry or deprived. Best of all, you won't need to hire a chef to make your meals palatable.

Likewise, the exercise component of the *Ten Years Thinner* program was specifically designed for sustainability. Although the routines described herein harness a groundbreaking physiological discovery, that doesn't mean that they are complicated, arduous, or even particularly time consuming. Each workout demands only a 20- to 25-minute daily time commitment and a very minimal level of initial fitness. Because they don't require any complicated exercise equip-ment or even a dedicated workout space, the routines can be done virtually any-where, anytime, and by anyone. Regardless of your current activity level, this home-friendly training program will stoke your metabolism to incinerate body fat more efficiently than if you spent hours marching away on a treadmill.

YOU ARE NOT "GOING ON A DIET"

The vast majority of so-called diets cater to our penchant for quick fixes. But when it comes to healthy eating, there is no such thing as a magic bullet. Fad diets that eliminate entire food groups and starvation diets that severely restrict calories contradict the basic machinery of human physiology. In the long run, these approaches are doomed to fail.

Although severe caloric restriction may lead to initial weight loss, the very nature of such an approach precludes its long-term effectiveness. Weight loss by caloric restriction triggers hormonal modifications that our species evolved to survive times of famine. These physiological mechanisms involve metabolic slowing, muscle wasting, exaggerated fat retention, and changes in brain chemistry that contribute to the development of behaviors like binge eating. The preferential loss of lean tissue (muscle) over fat often results in a false sense of accomplishment. You do lose weight. However, the "new you" is merely a smaller, flabbier version of the old you. Once normal eating patterns resume, the weight rapidly returns, plus an added ten pounds. Why? Because the muscle you sacrificed during the period of forced starvation, combined with metabolic slowing, make it that much harder for your body to burn fat.

THE MIRACLE OF MUSCLE

When it comes to having a firm, flab-free physique, have you ever noticed that many people are able to coast along on youth until they're about 20 or 25 years old? After that, without at least minimal attention to diet and exercise, body composition begins to deteriorate. The untended human physique will get softer and flabbier with every passing year. In fact, for many years, the medical community subscribed to the belief that decreases in metabolic rate and subsequent weight gain were "natural" and "unavoidable" consequences of aging. Well, I can assure you that's simply wrong! But before I dispel this myth, consider a little story I heard a long time ago called "Dr. Dents and the Frog."

Dr. Dents and the Frog

One day, a scientist named Dr. Dents decided to do an experiment. He went to the pond behind his laboratory and caught an old bullfrog. Then he took the frog back to his lab and put it on the table.

"*Jump!*" yelled Dr. Dents, and the startled frog jumped.

Dr. Dents opened his notebook and made the following entry: *frog jumps on command.* Then Dr. Dents cut a length of twine and tied the frog's two front legs together.

"*Jump!*" he yelled again, and again, the startled frog managed to jump. Dr. Dents wrote in his notebook: *with front legs bound, frog jumps on command.*

Then Dr. Dents cut another length of twine and hog tied the frog's back legs tightly to its front legs.

"*Jump!*" he yelled again, but this time the poor frog didn't move.

Excited by his discovery, Dr. Dents grabbed up his notebook and scribbled: *with all four legs bound, frog goes deaf.*

"Dr. Dents and the Frog" is my favorite parable for bad science. You might find it difficult to swallow that real-life researchers could be guilty of such obvious errors in judgment. Well, believe it or not, bad science happens all the time. Alas, even the world's most prestigious white coats, even the Harvard MD's and the Yale PhD's and the Stanford MD/PhD's and all the other impressive acronyms indigenous to various Meccas of academia, yes, even *they* have been known to draw unfounded conclusions from research data. Usually, bad science happens because of honest mistakes like poor study design, flawed methods of data collection, uncontrolled variables, and plain old human error. (Sometimes, however, bad science happens because researchers have *agendas*; remember, even so-called objective studies are funded by *someone*.)

Thanks to some (very bad) science, for many years, the medical community clung to the idea that weight gain was a natural and largely unavoidable consequence of aging. This view was based on research data that showed that most adults get fatter as they get older. Unfortunately, the study failed to account for a number of very important variables, including physical activity. Subsequent research has indicated that people don't really get fatter as a direct result of aging per se. They get fatter because, *as* they age, the vast majority of people *become less active*. As our friend Dr. Dents illustrated so eloquently, things are sometimes more complicated than they seem at first glance.

When researchers delved more deeply into the phenomenon of aging and weight gain, they discovered that most adults were not merely gaining body fat as they got older, they were also losing muscle mass. This fact alone has enormous bearing on why people tend to gain weight as they age.

Muscle is a very special tissue. In terms of metabolic activity, pound for pound, muscle tissue is second only to nervous (brain) tissue. In other words, it takes more calories to maintain a given volume of muscle tissue than the same volume of just about every other tissue in the entire human body. And because we possess many more pounds of muscle than any other tissue type, the vast majority of our daily caloric expenditure goes to using, repairing, and maintaining our muscles. This is true even if you lead a relatively sedentary existence. In fact, if you are currently sedentary, very marginal increases in muscle activity can greatly enhance caloric expenditure and fat burning. And if you are currently active, very modest increases in muscle mass will accomplish the same goal. In other words, the more toned you are, the more fat you will burn. Don't worry, you don't have to spend hours at the gym lifting weights to reap the benefits of a revved metabolism; a little extra muscle goes a surprisingly long way.

Additionally, the more muscle you possess, the higher your resting metabolic rate, and the more calories you will burn over time even if you're just lying around channel surfing. Of course, channel surfing is not the ideal way to accomplish muscle toning. The old adage "use it or lose it" is especially true when it comes to firm flesh. Adults who do not exercise regularly will typically lose between five and seven pounds of muscle mass every decade. To put this into perspective, a five-pound muscle loss translates to roughly 250 fewer calories burned each day. This can add up to over 25 pounds of fat gain in a *single year*!

How can you prevent this from happening to you? Simple! Adopt an exercise program designed to efficiently build and maintain adequate muscle to fuel around-the-clock fat burning. But is it really possible to *add* muscle *while* you shed body fat?

Intuitively, the idea seems to defy logic. After all, it takes an excess of calories to *build* tissue, and a caloric deficit to *lose* tissue. Right? Not entirely. Despite half a century of (good) science to the contrary, many people (including, unfortunately, many so-called weight loss experts) continue to view human metabolism like a bank account into which we deposit and withdraw calories like currency. The notion that you need to spend more calories than you consume in order to lose body fat is deceptive. Dozens of studies indicate that the appropriate dietary practices, coupled with regular exercise, will induce simultaneous muscle gain and fat loss—without counting calories. Physiologists are discovering that the *quality* of the calories you consume is far more important than the overall quantity. Likewise, the quality of the food is far more important than the food group to which it belongs. You will never have to sacrifice variety for good health, or good health for good looks. When it comes to nutrition, thankfully, they all go hand in hand.

NUTRITION 101:
A LESSON IN HOMEOSTASIS

Have you ever stopped to wonder why you need food to survive? It might seem fairly obvious, but the complete explanation is exceedingly complicated. In essence, however, it all boils down to *homeostasis*, which is really just a fancy word for physiological balance, or *equilibrium*. The more steadfast and unfaltering our overall homeostasis, the better our state of health.

From the moment we are conceived until the moment we draw our last breath, our life represents a glorious and (temporarily) successful battle against the most lethal force in the universe: *entropy*, the tendency towards chaos. Our very existence as living organisms relies on a precariously maintained balance between interdependent systems and processes. Should even a tiny component of this bewildering array of life-sustaining functions be thrown off-kilter, it damages our health and jeopardizes our ability to offset future disturbances.

The human body can compensate for a wide variety of assaults to homeostasis. However, each time our body engages to combat an ongoing threat to our health, our physiological equilibrium shifts to a new, less stable set point. The more chronic battles we must fight, the more the balance of life tips toward chaos. Eventually, we run out of ammunition. When our body can no longer defend itself against disequilibrium, we lose the war against entropy and draw our last breath.

Conceptually, you can think of homeostasis like an old-fashioned scale. However, instead of a single beam from which two pans are suspended, there are *millions* of beams suspended from millions of other beams, like an infinitely complicated child's mobile. Some of the beams are colossal; others are microscopic. And at both ends of every beam, regardless of its size or position, you will find a pair of pans.

Each time you add or subtract a weight from a pan on the scale of homeostasis, every single one of the millions of beams adjusts accordingly. While beams in closest proximity to the disturbance usually display the greatest movements, even the most remote beam will shift incrementally with the addition or removal of weight from any pan. To prevent pans from tipping, the scale requires a steady supply of both counterweights and a processing and distribution system for delivering the appropriate denominations of those counterweights to the areas where they are needed. In other words, to successfully maintain the complicated balancing act of homeostasis, the body requires a steady supply of both matter and energy. This is where food comes in.

To illustrate this point, let's consider your muscles. To be firm and toned, your muscles need the elemental building blocks of tissue growth. Muscle toning also requires energy to deliver the building blocks to the muscles, energy to direct the building blocks to where they are needed within the muscle fibers, and energy to remove damaged tissue and metabolic waste products. Not to mention the huge amounts of energy demanded by the very muscle contractions that made your physique firm in the first place. Small wonder that your muscles represent such a metabolically active region of your body!

Although you are capable of using all three basic macronutrients—protein, carbohydrate, and fat—as caloric energy sources, carbohydrate is your body's preferred fuel for muscle contraction. However, only protein can provide the building blocks your body needs for muscle growth and repair. In fact, the structural integrity of virtually all human tissue, from muscles, tendons, and ligaments to skin, hair, and organs, relies on a protein framework. In the gastrointestinal (GI) tract, dietary protein is broken down into molecular subunits, known as amino acids, which can then be reassembled to create new proteins according to your body's specific needs.

While it's true that fat can also make a structural contribution, especially toward padding your hips, thighs, and belly, excess fat accumulation usually represents an unneeded and unwelcome contribution. However, eliminating dietary fat from your meal plan is absolutely, positively, one hundred percent counterproductive to eliminating stored fat. As will become clear in the coming chapters, when your diet lacks sufficient amounts of the right kinds of fat, stored fat becomes largely inaccessible as an energy source. I think that bears repeating: If you don't eat fat, you won't burn fat.

One of the keys to fat loss is knowing which fats to eat, and which fats to avoid. Indeed, there are several distinct types of *fatty acid*, the molecular subunit of fat, and each impacts human physiology and homeostasis differently. Knowing the difference between them can spell the difference between a flabby body and a firm physique, between clogged arteries and clear ones, and between chronic disease and extended longevity.

In addition to the three fundamental macronutrients, your body also requires a staggering array of *micro*nutrients, including vitamins, minerals, and other trace elements. Micronutrient deficiencies can spell the demise of homeostasis, good health, and a firm physique.

Now that you have a basic understanding of *why* you need to eat in order to build a firm physique, I'd like to provide you with a better understanding of *how* you need to eat in order to hone your beautiful body. To put it simply, your success in the arena of physique firming is a direct reflection of your success in the battle against entropy (and disease). Like every other component of your physiology, good muscle health is inextricably linked to good health in general. And a diet that promotes a beautiful body and smooth skin is a diet that, by definition, also promotes optimal health. This is an extremely important point: Eating for a firm, youthful physique equals eating for optimal health, and vice versa.

THE LEAN ESSENTIALS:

- Food provides matter and energy for maintaining physiological equilibrium or homeostasis.

- The three basic macronutrients, protein, carbohydrate, and fat, can all be used as caloric energy sources.

- Carbohydrate is your body's preferred fuel for muscle contraction.

- Only protein can provide the building blocks your body needs for muscle growth and repair.

- You need to eat fat in order to burn fat.

- Eating for a firm, youthful physique also means eating for optimal health.

EVOLUTION:
THE ULTIMATE REALITY CHECK

When it comes to matters of health, an understanding of our own evolutionary history is perhaps the most powerful reality check we have at our disposal. I suspect that much of the current research pertaining to weight loss could be taken up a notch if investigators would bear that fact in mind when designing their experimental approaches. Rather than view the human genome as a stagnant entity, what if researchers were to remind themselves that our DNA tells a dynamic story spanning millions of years? A story that remains meticulously catalogued within our genes—if only we remember to look there!

The evolutionary process is based on the compassionless principal of natural selection. Although modern humans have only been around for about 50,000 years, the countless adaptations that contributed to our genetic makeup occurred over a period of *millions* of years. Those adaptations that gave us a survival advantage were passed on to succeeding generations. Those that did not were unceremoniously eliminated from the gene pool. As a result, modern humans have been physiologically, anatomically, and psychologically shaped by environmental pressures dating back to the dawn of time.

For example, climactic changes that occurred about 5 million years ago resulted in widespread deforestation which eventually led our primate ancestors to transition from tree-dwelling in the lush jungle to freestanding in the dry savannah. This entailed a tremendous shift in survival strategies. Terrestrial primates would have been faced with a plethora of difficult challenges—from decreases in readily available food sources to a greater vulnerability to predators. The subsequent adaptations that permitted our ancestors' survival shaped our development as a species.

The Caveman Diet

Archeological data indicate that 40,000 to 50,000 years ago, prehistoric men and women were tall, strapping athletes with defined muscles and very little body fat. They were fit, strong, and healthy. Forty thousand years ago, obesity and heart disease were nonexistent.

How did these hot-bodied prehistoric humans live? Early humans were hunter-gatherers who subsisted on a diet that was extremely high in animal-based food sources. For the majority of hunter-gatherer societies, an estimated two-thirds to three-quarters of their total caloric intake came from wild game. They also consumed significant amounts of plant matter in the form of fruits, tubers, leafy vegetation, nuts, and seeds. Compared to our modern North American diet, the Stone Age meal plan was higher in protein and lower in energy-dense carbohydrates.

Interestingly, although hunter-gatherer societies consumed what would now be considered unhealthy amounts of dietary fat, early humans were lean and muscular, and their arteries were free of the plaques that lead to heart disease and stroke. As predicted by natural selection, millions of years of evolution shaped hunter-gatherer physiology to thrive on the foods that early humans could reliably find in their environment.

Then, about 10,000 years ago, the pressures of increasing population density in many parts of Europe, Africa, and Asia forced an abrupt shift from the nomadic, hunter-gatherer lifestyle to more geographically stable populations that depended on agriculture for survival. The advent of civilization brought about the domestication of livestock and the introduction of dairy foods, as well as the cultivation of tubers and root vegetables, legumes, and cereal grains like rice, oats, and wheat.

After the advent of agriculture, and more specifically, the cultivation of grains, the human species lost a foot in height and experienced a significantly increased incidence of infections, anemia, bone disease, tooth defects, cavities, infant mortality, and a sizable reduction in life span.

Why did this happen? Because the dietary revolution that resulted from the switch to a cereal grain–based diet caused the introduction of numerous food items for which our genetic predisposition was not prepared. Until ten thousand years ago—a mere blink of an eye compared to our genetic life span—the environment that dictated our genetic makeup did not include grains. Unlike the birds, rodents, and grazers that are able to consume grains without suffering harmful effects, our ancestors, the primates, did not evolve in the savanna. We spent the first several million years of our evolutionary history in tropical forests eating an entirely different class of plant. As a result, we were never physiologically equipped to digest, absorb, and assimilate grains in a way that promotes a well-balanced homeostasis, a strong healthy body, or a firm, flab-free physique.

Anthropologists believe that our hasty shift to a grain-based diet, for which we were genetically ill prepared, lies at the root of many modern degenerative diseases, as well as the deterioration of our muscle mass in favor of fat storage. For starters, grains lack many essential vitamins and minerals. Moreover, certain components of many cereal grains interfere with the absorption of other vital nutrients. As grains began to displace nutrient-rich fruits and vegetables in the diet of our unsuspecting ancestors, humans became increasingly prone to vitamin deficiencies. And homeostasis does not take kindly to vitamin deficiencies! Malnutrition causes every precariously balanced, life-sustaining process to swing like a pendulum. And once our internal equilibrium begins to deteriorate, our health starts to decline.

In addition to their beggarly vitamin and mineral content, grains also harbor an unhealthy complement of essential fatty acids. While they are high in *linoleic acid*, which is the main precursor to omega-6 essential fatty acid production, grains are completely devoid of omega-3 essential fatty acids. As scientists have only recently discovered, a diet that includes too many omega-6 essential fatty acids or too few omega-3 essential fatty acids induces a homeostatic shift that favors the production of inflammatory compounds. In turn, an excess of inflammatory compounds promotes low-grade, widespread *inflammation* throughout the body.

INFLAMMATION: THE MOTHER OF MODERN DISEASE

In a nutshell, inflammation is the body's way of dealing with illness or injury. Inflammation allows blood to clot, injured tissue to heal, and devitalized tissue to be cleared away. Inflammation seeks out abnormal cells and dispatches them. Inflammation also attacks foreign invaders like bacteria, viruses, and parasites, and either destroys them or battles to keep them in check. Without inflammation, we would bleed to death from every paper cut; we would develop multiple malignant tumors on a daily basis; and the first time we caught a cold would also be our last. The ability to mount an inflammatory response is a critical part of human immunity and is absolutely necessary to our survival.

So far, inflammation sounds like a pretty good thing to have a lot of. So what's the big deal if our grain-based diet contains extra omega-6 essential fatty acids and not so many omega-3's? Until just a few years ago, scientists didn't think it was all that big a deal either. Oh how times have changed!

The more researchers explore the mechanisms of illness, the more they are discovering that overzealous inflammation lies at the root of just about every modern disease process known to man. Everything from diabetes to heart disease, autoimmune disorders, depression, osteoporosis, Alzheimer's, allergies, skin disorders, infertility, digestive disorders, cancer, obesity, and even *aging* is now being traced back to maladaptive inflammation.

As with every other process that contributes to life-sustaining homeostasis, healthy inflammatory responses rely on a delicate balance between two opposing forces. The yin and yang of inflammation are pro-inflammatory compounds and anti-inflammatory compounds. Unfortunately, many aspects of modern living, including our diet, are proving to be exceedingly pro-inflammatory. As the balance shifts further and further toward this extreme, humans become increasingly prone to obesity, diabetes, heart disease, and premature aging.

Taking Responsibility

Although we write sonnets, erect skyscrapers, explore outer space, and transplant organs, anatomically and physiologically our bodies are relics of the Stone Age. The things early humans ate and thrived on fifteen, twenty, thirty, forty, and fifty thousand years ago are the same things that make us healthiest today. Millions of years of environmental pressures and natural selection determined our bodies' nutritional requirements. We are remarkably arrogant to think that we can deny our genetic heritage without incurring the wrath of evolution. Oh, we can ignore our genes all right. But they will not ignore us!

Alas, the preagricultural Stone Age was a wondrous period: a time when humans did not have to worry about eating a "healthy diet." Realistically, they had very little choice in the matter; all the foods that were readily available to our prehistoric ancestors were healthy for them to eat. We, on the other hand, are not so fortunate. The vast majority of the foods that are readily available for our consumption do NOT promote good health *or* a firm physique. On the contrary, most of the items lining today's grocery store aisles promote disease, premature aging, and a flabby physique. But *we* have something that our Stone Age counterparts did not: *We* have the power to make a choice about what we put into our bodies.

But with power comes responsibility.

Once you possess the knowledge for restoring homeostasis and building a fabulous, youthful physique, you owe it to your health, and your self-esteem, to do so.

THE LEAN ESSENTIALS:

- Foods that were good for us 10,000 years ago are the same foods that are good for us today.

- Many aspects of modern living, including most dietary practices, are highly pro-inflammatory.

- A pro-inflammatory diet contributes to chronic disease, obesity, and the cosmetic signs of aging.

————— ❯❯❯❯❯ —————

"I've never liked how my pants fit me because I've always
had these bulges on the side of my hips. Thanks to the
Ten Years Thinner program the bulges are gone.
Now I love how I look in my clothes!" — COLLEEN, 43

"Not only do I have the body I have wanted for a long time,
but I also have the metabolism I need to maintain it." — JILLIAN, 38

"My body shape is so different since I started doing the
Ten Years Thinner program, I'm always getting asked
how much weight I've lost. I try to explain how muscle weighs
more than fat and takes up less volume, but most people just
don't get it. The other day I got out my bag of 'skinny' clothes,
the stuff I used to wear 10 years ago, before I had kids.
The fitted tops and pants were all too big for me—even though
I weigh the same now as I did then!" — DARLENE, 43

————— ❮❮❮❮❮ —————

CHAPTER 2

Protein for Pulverizing Paunch

Despite what you might have seen on TV, you cannot lounge your belly fat into oblivion, squeeze your way to thinner thighs, or massage yourself a perkier fanny any more than you can wish your way to Wonderland. In the vast and mysterious realm of physique sculpting, there is no such thing as fairy dust: Spot reduction is a fallacy, a farce, a big FAT lie.

Fat accumulates on your body in a pattern determined by a combination of hormonal factors, genetics, gender, and age. You will ordinarily lose body fat in the reverse order that you put it on. No matter how many sit-ups, crunches, slides, squeezes, squashes, and rolls you do, you cannot target a problem area for fat loss. Stimulating the muscle beneath the flab will not dissipate the flab, it will simply tone the underlying muscle. Of course, toning the muscle causes the muscle to grow, which ultimately stimulates fat burning.

But doesn't "tone" mean that you're *adding* muscle? And if your main objective is to reduce your size, isn't *adding* more muscle counterproductive to your physique goals?

NOT AT ALL!

The muscle you add will increase your metabolic rate, which, in turn, will devour the fat from every part of your body. Plus, muscle is three times as dense as fat. In other words, one pound of fat occupies three times as much volume as one pound of muscle. What does this mean in the context of building your dream physique? Think of it this way: If you were to exchange every pound of flab surrounding your hips, thighs, and buttocks for a pound of muscle, even though you wouldn't lose any weight per se, your hips, thighs, and buttocks would lose about half their volume. Without losing any weight at all, you could transform jiggly hips, cottage cheese thighs, and a saggy fanny into firm hips, defined thighs, and a perky posterior.

Moreover, every extra ounce of muscle you carry stokes your metabolic rate, which, in turn, burns your fat. Current estimates indicate that every pound of muscle an individual possesses devours between 35 and 75 calories per day *simply to exist*—and that doesn't even include the calories your muscles burn during physical activity. For every three pounds of muscle gained by the average individual, resting metabolic rate increases by 7 percent, and daily caloric requirements increase by 15 percent.

Muscle toning equals fat burning!

Obviously, the more muscle you possess, the more fat you will burn. Unfortunately, the billions of dollars spent marketing abdominal devices as the key to fat loss have many late-night television viewers convinced that you can crunch, lounge, roll, and slide your way to a glorious physique. In actuality, because your abs represent such a small fraction of your total muscle mass, exclusively targeting your abdominal muscles to induce fat loss is like trying to extinguish a forest fire with a garden hose.

Doesn't it make more sense to implement a full-body routine that works all your muscles? Especially the larger muscle groups comprising your thighs, butt, shoulders, and back? By virtue of their large size, your quads, hamstrings, glutes, delts, pecs, and lats are veritable fat-burning factories. Contracting these muscles requires substantial energy expenditure and burns loads of calories. More significantly, every ounce of toned muscle you possess incrementally raises your metabolic rate for around-the-clock fat burning. Put simply, by toning your muscles, you are implementing a vigorous fat-burning program for your entire body! And rest assured, the exercise routines described in upcoming chapters *will* melt fat faster and more efficiently than any other workout you have ever tried.

When it comes to building toned muscles, exercise is only part of the equation. For best results, you will also need to adopt a meal plan that simultaneously supports muscle development and diverts fat storage. In this respect, adequate dietary protein is absolutely crucial. Indeed, protein tops the list as the most important macronutrient in your muscle-toning arsenal.

THE LEAN ESSENTIALS:

- Spot reduction is a big FAT lie; you can't *target* specific fat deposits for shrinkage.

- Muscle is three times as dense as fat. Hence, one pound of fat occupies three times as much space as one pound of muscle.

- Every pound of muscle an individual possesses devours between 35 and 75 calories per day.

- *Muscle toning equals fat burning!* Every ounce of toned muscle you possess increases around-the-clock fat burning.

- Protein is the most important macronutrient in your muscle-toning arsenal.

THE NUTS AND BOLTS OF PROTEIN

What is protein?

As I touched on in Chapter 1, protein is one of the three basic macronutrients comprising the foods we eat. (The remaining two are fat and carbohydrate.) On a molecular level, protein consists of long chains of nitrogen-containing subunits known as amino acids. Of the 21 different amino acids that go into building a protein chain, nine of them are considered *essential amino acids* because the human body lacks the physiological machinery to assemble them from their component parts. Of the remaining twelve amino acids, three of them are considered to be *conditionally essential* because, in many instances, our bodies become too overwhelmed to assemble them in sufficient quantities.

You do not have to know the names or recognize the different structures of the various amino acids to grasp the significance of adequate protein intake. However, it is important to appreciate that over half of all amino acids cannot be manufactured by the body in sufficient quantities to promote muscle toning, and that adequate amounts of these amino acids *must* be included in the diet. (I will elaborate on this concept later in the chapter.)

Although proteins contain four calories per gram, they do not ordinarily serve as primary fuel sources. Instead, proteins are the main building blocks of virtually every living animal tissue. The structural integrity of the human body, from tendons and ligaments to muscles and organs, relies on a protein framework. To maintain, repair, or add to existing tissues, the body must synthesize genetically defined protein configurations. Although this principle applies to virtually all tissues, adequate protein intake is especially important for maintaining muscle mass.

Unlike your internal organs, which are surrounded and protected by your rib cage, pelvis, and skull, peripheral organs like skin and muscle are more vulnerable to environmental stressors. Our skin acts as a physical barrier between us and the outside world. It is our first line of defense against insect bites, burns, infectious agents, radiation, allergens, sharp objects, blunt force, friction, and countless other potentially damaging assaults. Although our muscles must also contend with many of these same dangers, the greatest source of muscle trauma is actually muscle use. Physical exertion causes microscopic damage, known as *microtrauma*, within muscle fibers. It takes a steady supply of raw materials to repair and maintain healthy skin and muscle.

So, if you want both vibrant, young-looking skin and a firm, toned physique, you must provide your body with ample amounts of high-quality protein. By "high quality," I mean protein that contains a significant compliment of essential (and conditionally essential) amino acids. Protein foods that derive from animal sources, such as dairy products, eggs, poultry, meat, and fish, are rich in essential amino acids. These foods are also great sources of nitrogen, which is integral to the synthesis of many important compounds including nonessential amino acids.

THE FATE OF
DIETARY PROTEIN

During digestion, proteins consumed in the diet are broken down by the mechanical process of chewing. Once the food is swallowed and reaches the stomach and intestines, enzymes known as *proteases* go to work on proteins to further reduce them into microscopic particles of protein or *peptides*, as well as individual amino acids. Amino acids and small peptides are absorbed into the bloodstream directly through the intestinal walls. Once they enter the general circulation, these tiny bits of protein are typically captured by cells of different tissues and used in the construction of new protein chains. However, during times of intense physical activity, like a physique-firming exercise routine, blood-born amino acids are grabbed up by the liver, where they are stripped of their nitrogen component (a process known as *deamination*) and chemically converted to glucose (a form of carbohydrate) for energy.

In other words, the fate of amino acids is determined by the body's needs. When caloric intake is ample, ingested protein is earmarked for the growth, repair, and maintenance of tissues like skin and muscle. On the other hand, when caloric intake falls short of the body's requirements, amino acids can also be used as a calorie-generating energy source. Because amino acids are the building blocks of your soon-to-be firm physique, the fate of the protein you eat has far-reaching implications in terms of body composition.

Optimal muscle toning—which, as you now know, contributes to maximal fat burning—requires a steady supply of amino acids. When caloric restriction necessitates the diversion of amino acids for glucose production, your muscles get shortchanged. By depriving your muscles of the basic materials needed for growth and repair, you not only prevent them from reaching their full, firm potential, you also prevent optimal fat burning.

Even if your diet includes sufficient calories to fulfill your body's energy requirements, without adequate dietary protein and a steady supply of essential amino acids, muscle tissue suffers. Remember, virtually every tissue in the human body relies on amino acid building blocks for growth and repair. In addition, there are numerous other nitrogen-containing compounds essential to human life including DNA, RNA, hormones, pigments like melanin, and heme, the oxygen-carrying component of red blood cells.

As you might recall from Chapter 1, your body perceives nutritional deficiencies as a threat to your life-sustaining homeostasis; every system in your body will do whatever is necessary to avert the threat to your physiological equilibrium. As far as your body is concerned, the manufacture of vital hormones and blood components is more important than toning your muscles. When dietary protein is lacking, your body will cannibalize its own muscle tissue to create a steady supply of amino acids for the maintenance of internal organs and the manufacture of vital compounds. Your body is more than happy to sacrifice your firm physique in order to stay alive. However, from the standpoint of a revved metabolism and increased fat burning, muscle breakdown is the kiss of death!

Which brings me back to a concept I introduced in Chapter 1: simultaneous muscle toning and fat burning. I realize the whole idea seems counterintuitive. After all, it takes an excess of calories and amino acid building blocks to tone muscle and a shortage of calories to shed fat. How is it possible to have both processes occurring simultaneously? The key to this physiological paradox lies in the *type* of caloric surplus you create. In essence, you can still induce a fat-burning energy deficit even if your diet includes a protein surplus.

In times of energy restriction, your body will liberate stored fat as a source of needed calories. True, your body will also sacrifice some muscle tissue to generate calories. However, provided there is an adequate surplus of protein in your diet, your body is actually able to build new muscle tissue faster than it gets torn down. Hence your body is capable of adding to your existing muscle mass *while* you shed your existing fat mass.

Wait a minute: Protein contains four calories per gram. If it takes an *excess* of protein to support muscle development, how is it possible to create an energy *deficit* with a surplus of dietary protein? What happens to the "extra calories" from increased protein intake? Can "too much" protein make you fat?

Not likely!

First, protein digestion requires significant energy expenditure in and of itself. The consumption of a high protein meal measurably raises your body temperature and metabolic rate, a process known as *thermogenesis*. And second, in order for ingested protein to be stored as fat, it must first be converted to glucose, a process that requires high levels of the hormone *glucagon* relative to the hormone *insulin*. This hormonal ratio only occurs when an individual is in the "starved" state, i.e., they have not eaten for at least four or five hours. In order for your body to then covert the glucose to fat, high levels of insulin relative to glucagon must be present. This hormonal ratio only occurs when an individual is in the fed state. Because it is virtually impossible for these hormonal situations to co-exist, it is virtually impossible for your body to store excess protein calories as fat!

This is the single most important governing principle behind the initial success of every high-protein diet, program, and product in existence. Notice I said "initial." The long-term viability of an eating plan, i.e., whether or not you can tolerate it over time, whether or not it will continue to produce the desired effects, and whether or not it is ultimately a healthy diet, depends largely on the two remaining macronutrients, fat and carbohydrate.

THE LEAN ESSENTIALS:

- Protein, which consists of long chains of amino acid subunits, is the main building block of virtually every tissue in our bodies, including muscle.

- If dietary protein is lacking, your body will cannibalize its own muscle tissue to create a steady supply of amino acids for the maintenance of internal organs and the manufacture of vital compounds.

- From the standpoint of a revved metabolism and decreased body fat, muscle breakdown is the kiss of death!

- While it is possible to add muscle while you burn fat, it is virtually impossible for your body to store excess protein calories as fat.

PROTEIN INTAKE:
HOW MUCH, HOW OFTEN, AND FROM WHAT?

By now, you are probably wondering just how much protein you need to consume in order to create a muscle-toning, fat-burning, protein surplus. Luckily, there's some (good) science behind the answers to questions like these.

Not surprisingly, individuals who exercise regularly have greater nutritional requirements than people who are sedentary. This principle applies to both *micronutrients* (vitamins, minerals, and trace elements) and *macronutrients* (protein, fat, and carbohydrate). There are several major reasons why active people have increased protein requirements.

First, exercise doesn't just burn extra calories, it also breaks down muscle tissue. Physical exertion causes microscopic damage, known as *microtrauma*, within muscle fibers. It takes both fuel, in the form of calories, and raw materials, in the form of amino acids, to repair this damage. Second, your muscle fibers adapt to a training challenge by becoming bigger and stronger. As with muscle repair, muscle growth or *hypertrophy* requires an increased supply of both fuel and raw materials. And third, as discussed previously, muscle is an extremely metabolically active tissue. Your body needs a constant supply of calories and amino acids just to maintain your muscle. Any increase to your total muscle mass calls for more of both.

Studies that explore the protein requirements of active people have yielded some surprising results. For optimal muscle retention and toning, research indicates that people who participate in regular endurance activities like jogging and cycling need about 1.3 grams of protein per kilogram of body weight per day; those involved in resistance training need about 1.7 grams per kilogram of body weight per day.

The *Ten Years Thinner* exercise routine incorporates aspects of both cardiovascular exercise and light strength training for the fastest results possible. In other words, the workout represents a blending of endurance and resistance training. For best results, you should eat somewhere between 1.3 and 1.7 grams of protein per kilogram of ideal body weight per day, or roughly three-quarters of a gram of protein per pound of ideal body weight per day. In other words, if your target weight is around 120 pounds, you would want to be eating around .75 x 120 = 90 grams of protein per day. This is equivalent to the amount of protein found in 15 eggs, *or* 4 chicken breasts, *or* 3 cans of tuna fish.

That's a lot of protein!

Not surprisingly, most active people don't consume anywhere near the amount of protein they need for optimal muscle toning and fat burning. And unfortunately, merely getting enough protein does not guarantee that you will optimize muscle toning. When it comes to protein, *how often* you eat is just as important as *how much* you eat. Because the body is unable to store excess protein, it must be ingested every two to three hours to provide a constant supply of amino acids for muscle growth, maintenance, and repair.

Choosing the right types of protein is also important. For simultaneous muscle toning and fat burning, lean animal protein sources are best because animal protein is the most "complete" form of protein. While it's possible to obtain all of the essential amino acids on a vegan diet, only animal protein contains all 21 amino acids in the ratios that approximate human muscle tissue.

To illustrate this concept, imagine that you have a box that contains one of every letter of the alphabet. In other words, you have the complete alphabet. If you wanted to spell MUSCLE, you would have no problem. But if you wanted to spell FIRM MUSCLE, you could run into difficulties after the first "M." Being clever, it might occur to you to take the "W" and turn it upside down for the second "M."

Your body is very clever when it comes to creating protein chains from available amino acids. In fact, your body is capable of creating all twelve *non-essential* amino acids by rearranging the structures of other amino acids. But what about the remaining nine *essential* amino acids?

Back to our alphabet box analogy, if you wanted to spell TIGHT MUSCLE, you wouldn't be able to do it because there's only one "T" in your box of letters, and there are no letters that you can flip or turn sideways to make resemble a "T." The nine essential amino acids are like the letter "T." Even if your letter box (diet) contains all 26 letters (includes all 21 amino acids), there will be many words (proteins) that you simply cannot spell (that your body cannot synthesize). As a result, your letter-box vocabulary (your physique-firming potential) will be severely limited (will never be realized).

It's extremely difficult to obtain adequate concentrations of essential amino acids from plant protein sources, even so-called complete protein foods like tofu. In fact, it's essentially impossible to optimize muscle growth and retention on a vegan diet. Lacto-ovo vegetarians tend to fare better than vegans because their diets permit the consumption of dairy products and eggs.

Accordingly, the *Ten Years Thinner* meal plan calls for a minimum amount of animal-based protein with each of your three meals. Although there is a wide variety of protein foods to choose from (and an infinite number of recipes you can create using these foods), lean protein sources like skinless chicken, game, and seafood are recommended over fatty cuts of poultry, red meat, and pork.

The reasons for this are not solely because of the high calorie content of fat. In the latter half of the 1800s, the "science" of fattening cattle as rapidly and excessively as possible made great strides. By the mid-1880s, feedlots were generating obese, 1,200-pound steers in barely two years. Nowadays, modern feedlots can perform this magic in just 14 months! There is one problem though: It appears that the meat from animals force-fed a grain-based diet has a vastly different fat content than the flesh of the wild game we are genetically built to eat. Compared to domestic beef, similar cuts from wild deer and buffalo contain only about one-tenth the amount of total fat and saturated fat. Moreover, the fat of wild game exhibits four times as many omega-3 essential fatty acids as beef fat. It turns out that the omega-6 to omega-3 ratio of feedlot beef is highly pro-inflammatory.

As you know from Chapter 1, if your body is waging war against inflammation, it will negatively impact homeostasis, good health, and body composition. As far as your body is concerned, having a lean, youthful appearance is low on the totem pole of priorities. Maintaining life-sustaining homeostasis will always trump building a firm physique. If your body is distracted by inflammation, your physique will suffer.

One final word before we bid farewell to protein: If you are concerned about the potential health risks associated with increased protein intake, rest assured, there are none. A stockpile of research indicates that healthy individuals on high protein diets are not at any increased risk for health problems. Remember, our bodacious prehistoric ancestors consumed a diet that was two to three times higher in protein than the typical modern diet that is making us flabby and giving us heart disease. In fact, the scientific literature does not contain a single study to support the notion that high protein eating is bad for you. On the contrary, elevated protein intake doesn't just tone your muscles; it has also been linked to improved immune function, increased bone density, younger-looking skin, and decreased body fat.

THE LEAN ESSENTIALS:

- Active people have increased protein requirements.

- For a firm, youthful physique, you should eat roughly three fists' worth of protein per day.

- For simultaneous muscle toning and fat burning, lean animal protein sources are best.

- In addition to optimal muscle toning, adequate dietary protein has also been linked to improved immune function, increased bone density, younger-looking skin, and decreased body fat.

———— ❧❧❧❧❧ ————

"I was motivated to try *Ten Years Thinner* after learning
I had high cholesterol. I followed the program for six weeks and,
without medication, my cholesterol levels fell to well
within the normal range." — DEANNE, 35

"I started noticing subtle changes in my body
after two weeks, and HUGE changes after four. For the first
time in my adult life, I'm actually comfortable wearing
sleeveless shirts and tank tops!" — DARLENE, 43

"*Ten Years Thinner* runs on common sense, not guilt." — JILLIAN, 38

———— ❧❧❧❧❧ ————

CHAPTER 3

Fat for a Fabulous Physique

So, you thought eating fat would make you fat?

Well, you're in good company. Most of America still clings to the notion that fat in your diet makes you gain weight and gives you heart disease. It was exactly this brand of impaired logic that led to the low-fat diet scourge of the eighties. The decade that was responsible for MTV also spawned eating habits that irreparably damaged our health as a nation. More than a quarter of a century later, the repercussions of low-fat eating can still be felt in our collective subconscious. We are a nation of fat-phobes. Ironically, our fear of fat has played a massive role in making us the fattest population in the history of the planet.

Perhaps not surprisingly, it was a pile of bad science and politics (which has no business in science) that paved the way for the decade of diet disasters I casually refer to as the fat-free eighties. The low-fat eating movement got a leg up in 1977 after a Senate committee led by Senator George McGovern published its nutritional treatise entitled *Dietary Goals for the United States*. While McGovern admitted that he was "Faced with conflicting scientific opinions," he rationalized that "many of our health problems are sufficiently pressing that action has to be taken even if all scientific evidence is not in."

To be fair to the McGovern committee, many of their recommendations were actually quite reasonable. For example, they called for food labeling so consumers would know exactly what they were putting into their bodies. The committee advocated cutting back on red meat in favor of more poultry and fish, and recommended decreasing the amounts of sugar in our diet and increasing the amounts of fruits and vegetables. But then, unfortunately, they went a little too far. Essentially, *Dietary Goals for the United States* declared war on fat. McGovern's committee blamed our nation's increasing health care costs on an epidemic of "killer diseases" they figured were provoked by our unrestrained lust for lipids.

The McGovern committee's poor example of "taking action" despite a lack of scientific certainty was quickly followed by the prestigious National Institutes of Health (NIH). Indeed, the low-fat eating movement gained significant momentum in the early eighties when research conducted by the NIH reported an association between high blood cholesterol levels and an increased risk for heart attacks. Study authors reasoned that since dietary fat contained cholesterol, a good way to prevent heart attacks would be to encourage people to eat less fat. Ignorant of the physiological complexities of the nutritional issues they had only just begun to explore—remember Dr. Dents with his bullfrog experiment?—the experts at the National Institutes of Health made unsubstantiated assumptions about the data at hand and proceeded to jump to erroneous conclusions.

Senator McGovern was just a politician. But the distinguished scientists at the NIH really should have known better. Nevertheless, based on a small amount of largely conflicting research data, the NIH made an official recommendation that everyone over the age of two reduce their dietary fat intake. Then, after broadcasting their official recommendation, the NIH squandered hundreds of millions of tax dollars in an attempt to validate it. But no matter how much money the NIH poured into the research, they could never get the results to come out the way they wanted.

Months stretched into years, and still, study after expensive study failed to reveal a clear correlation between eating less fat and being thinner and healthier. Despite a complete lack of scientific evidence to support that reduced-fat eating induced either sustainable weight loss or lowered a person's risk for heart disease, the American Heart Association continues, to this day, to spawn version after version of those low-fat dietary abominations known as the food pyramids. But none of the low-fat, low-calorie diet models first popularized in the eighties do a single thing to make America thin and healthy. On the contrary, they have made us fatter and sicker than ever before!

Between 1960 and 1979, the prevalence of obesity among American adults climbed a paltry 1 percent. That's correct: During the twenty-year span that predated the fat-free eighties, the number of obese Americans went from 13 out of every 100 individuals to 14 out of every 100 individuals. Then, during the fat-free eighties, obesity among American adults soared by eight percentage points, reaching just over 22 percent by 1989. Today, 65 percent of American adults are considered overweight, and just over 35 out of every 100 American adults are classified as medically obese.

How do these figures translate in terms of our health as a nation? Put simply, nearly two-thirds of Americans are at an increased risk of developing high blood pressure, diabetes, cardiovascular disease, cancer, and arthritis as a direct result of their weight. Many of these same individuals will also encounter job discrimination and social rejection, suffer from low self-esteem and depression, and die prematurely.

In essence, America is being consumed by an obesity pandemic that teed off—more than 25 years ago—with the advent of low-fat diets. Coincidence? I think not!

Is it possible that the McGovern committee fingered the wrong villain? Rather than building sensible food pyramids, has the American Heart Association been erecting leaning towers of pizza (pun intended) for more than two decades? Has the NIH been asking the wrong question all along? Stay tuned to find out!

Perhaps it's time to refer back to our great reality check and consider our evolution as a species. According to anthropologists, 99.99 percent of our genetic makeup was already in place before the advent of agriculture. Hence, from a physiological perspective, we are still very much hunter-gatherers. For millions of years, the pressures of natural selection shaped our bodies to flourish on fat. Based on fossil evidence, carbon dating, energy expenditure research, and studies of surviving hunter-gatherer societies, anthropologists estimate that our ancestors consumed a diet that derived about 40 percent of its calories from fat sources. That's one-third more fat than the very upper limits of what is currently recommended by the American Heart Association as a healthy fat intake. Yet, as we discussed in Chapter 1, hunter-gatherers were hard-bodied athletes with no heart disease.

Where dietary fat is concerned, maybe it was never a question of *how much*. Maybe the hundred million dollar question should have been *what kinds*.

THE SKINNY ON THE
SLIMMING EFFECTS OF FAT

At 9 calories per gram, fat is the most energy dense of the three macronutrients. Gram for gram, fat contains more than twice the calories found in either protein or carbohydrate. But despite its high calorie content, dietary fat does not make you fat. In fact, current research indicates that the exact opposite is true—that you need to *eat* fat in order to *burn* fat. Although scientists continue to debate the biochemistry behind this apparent paradox, one thing is clear: If all other variables are held constant, including total caloric intake, overweight individuals who consume more fat relative to carbohydrate not only shed more pounds, but are better able to maintain their weight loss over time.

When it comes to a firm physique, dietary fat isn't just good for fat burning. As ingested fat arrives in your stomach, it causes the release of a hormone known as *cholecystokinin* (CCK). In turn, CCK signals your brain's satiety center that you have had enough to eat. By contributing to a subjective feeling of fullness, fat actually helps prevent overeating. In addition, fat retards the absorption of carbohydrate and protein from your gastrointestinal tract into your systemic circulation. In essence, the fat content of your meal prolongs your body's opportunity to utilize ingested food as an immediate fuel source. This reduces the likelihood that calories will spill over and wind up as unwanted fatty deposits.

In order to help promote a revved metabolism, prevent overeating, and divert fat storage, a healthy, physique-firming meal plan calls for the inclusion of fat with every single meal. But not just any fat will do. The types of fat you choose to make part of your diet have an important impact on both your body composition and your health. Eating the right kinds of fat can spell the difference between a flabby body and a toned physique, between clogged arteries and clear ones, and between chronic disease and extended longevity.

Indeed, fat's many talents extend far beyond promoting leanness. Adequate dietary fat is also crucial to countless physiological processes that contribute to a balanced homeostasis. Your body needs fat for proper absorption of vital nutrients and oxygen transport, for neurological health, cardiovascular health, reproductive health, for healthy skin and hair, and for robust immune function.

As you know, when any aspect of life-sustaining equilibrium is upset, even the smallest disturbance can have a far-reaching impact on other processes. In other

Oh Canada!

Perhaps one of the saddest things about American nutrition policy is that it refuses to remain contained within its borders. After the United States government maligned dietary fat in general and made saturated fat public enemy number one, the antifat movement spilled beyond geographical boundaries to influence eating habits around the globe. A quarter century later, our species is in the throes of a worldwide obesity pandemic.

Admittedly, the current state of affairs cannot be attributed entirely to American policy; part of the problem lies with the trappings of increasing industrialization. Motorized transit, sedentary occupations, and leisure activities that require nothing more than a couch and an opposable thumb all contribute to the declining muscle mass, energy expenditure, and metabolic rate that promote weight gain and heart disease. However, it is certainly plausible that an even more significant part of the problem relates to the widely held misconception that fat, in general, and saturated fat, in particular, are unhealthy and should be avoided at all costs. The health consequences of this blundered thinking are clearly exemplified by our friendly neighbors to the north.

When the United States declared war on fat in the late seventies and saturated fat in the early eighties, Canada became an ally, and the health repercussions for Canadians were catastrophic. According to a Canada Health Survey that was administered between 1977 and 1978, only 13.8 percent of Canadian adults were obese when Senator McGovern published his infamous treatise, *Dietary Goals for the United States*. Since then, just as it has done in the United States, the prevalence of obesity in Canada has skyrocketed at an unprecedented rate. According to the results of the most recent Canadian Community Health Survey, just over 23 percent of Canadian adults were obese as of 2004 and the number of obese children and teens had nearly tripled.

Despite the disheartening statistics, Canada's nutritional recommendations continue to mirror those of the United States. A quick perusal of Canada's Food Guide to Healthy Eating reveals that it is nothing more than a thinly veiled version of the American Heart Association's ghastly food pyramid. But Canada hasn't been an innocent pawn in these proceedings; Canada didn't simply join the fight against saturated fat, Canada fueled it with an elegant feat of genetic engineering that resulted in the first canola plant. Canola oil is now ubiquitous throughout the processed food industry, both in North America and abroad. But as it turns out, canola oil is anything but a healthy alternative to saturated fat. (We will revisit canola oil on page 49.)

words, if your fat intake were to fall short of your basic requirements for good health, your body would have to ration its supply of incoming fat in favor of processes that are most essential for your continued existence. For example, things like keeping your brain cells alive might take priority over more aesthetic concerns like firm, youthful skin or shiny hair. In most cases, if your body were forced to choose between keeping your face wrinkle-free or keeping your gray matter firing, your brain would get first dibs on nutrients, and that includes fat.

Fatty acids, the fundamental structural subunits of fat, act as hormonal modulators. Since hormones control virtually every vital physiological function, both adequate amounts *and* the correct balance of fatty acids are necessary for the properly harmonized operation of every single system in our body. Think of it this way: If amino acids are the body's construction materials, fatty acids are the body's communication system. And as with amino acids, certain fatty acids are considered *essential* because the human body lacks the ability to assemble them from raw materials. For optimal health and fat burning, your diet must include adequate amounts of essential fatty acids.

All fatty acid molecules contain carbon, hydrogen, and oxygen. Their basic structure consists of a chain of carbon atoms with an acid group stuck on one end. Most of the carbon atoms in the chain are joined together by a single chemical bond. Once in a while, carbon atoms are instead joined by double bonds. It is possible to modify the original structure of a fatty acid through various chemical processing techniques. For example, if a fatty acid contains a double bond between two of its carbon atoms, the process of *hydrogenation* can break the double bond, leaving a single-bond intact. To compensate for the loss of the bond, each carbon atom will grab an extra hydrogen atom. It is important to note that by altering the molecular structure of the fatty acid, these processing techniques significantly change how the fatty acid affects homeostasis.

THE LEAN ESSENTIALS:

- You need to eat fat in order to *burn* fat.

- Not only does fat make you feel full faster, it also slows the absorption of other macronutrients, decreasing the likelihood that calories will "spill over" and get stored as fat.

- *Fatty acids*, the fundamental subunits of fat, act as hormonal modulators. Just as amino acids function as the body's construction materials, fatty acids function as the body's messengers.

FATTY ACIDS
FOR A FIRM PHYSIQUE

From your body's perspective, there are four fundamental fatty acid subtypes.

Saturated Fatty Acids: OK in Moderation

Saturated fatty acids, which are solid at room temperature, are found, to some extent, in all animal protein sources. There are no double bonds between any neighboring carbon atoms in a saturated fatty acid. Because their carbon chains do not contain double bonds, saturated fatty acids are extremely stable and are not generally affected by industrial processing techniques. In other words, it is impossible to hydrogenate a saturated fatty acid because all the carbon atoms are already "saturated" with hydrogen.

Saturated fatty acids are found in high concentrations in meat fat, poultry skin, and dairy products like cheese and butter. As a fatty acid subclass, saturated fat has undergone conspicuous vilification over the past thirty years because of its alleged connection to obesity and heart disease. Although a diet that is high in saturated fat may raise total cholesterol, some researchers contend that there is little direct evidence linking saturated fat to either weight gain or heart disease. According to several extensive reviews of existing research data, statistically speaking, saturated fat in and of itself does not appear to make us flabbier, nor does it appear to raise our risk for a cardiac event. The debate continues.

While the scientists are busy duking it out over the questionable merits of saturated fat, we can take a lesson from our firm-bodied forefathers. Early humans consumed a diet that was loaded with animal protein, which, as you know, is the best dietary source of essential amino acids for promoting a firm, flab-free physique. Although the hunter-gatherer diet included large quantities of animal protein, the wild game available to Stone Age humans was many times leaner and contained only a fraction of the saturated fat of modern-day livestock.

Using evolution as the ultimate reality check, it seems clear that the most logical approach to a robust homeostasis, a healthy heart, and a revved metabolism for a lean physique is to limit our consumption of saturated fat without compromising the quantity or quality of essential amino acids in our diet. This means adopting a meal plan that emphasizes animal protein from leaner sources like skim milk, wild game, skinless poultry, seafood, and meat trimmed of all visible fat.

Monounsaturated Fatty Acids: The Fabbest of the Fats

If the carbon chain of a fatty acid contains at least one double bond, it is said to be "unsaturated." *Mono*unsaturated fats contain only one double bond; hence they are unsaturated at only one point within the carbon chain. Wherever a double bond occurs within the fatty acid, the carbon chain tends to kink. Because monounsaturated fatty acids are bent at odd angles, they will not lie next to each other in an orderly fashion like saturated fats. As a result, they solidify at a lower temperature than saturated fats and usually exist as liquids (oils) at room temperature.

Monounsaturated fatty acids are found in high concentrations in olives and olive oil, flaxseeds and flaxseed oil, peanuts and peanut oil, true nuts and nut oils, and avocados. Ongoing research indicates that diets that include increased amounts of monounsaturated fat, relative to both carbohydrate and other forms of fat, are better for promoting leaner body composition.

In addition, a rapidly expanding stockpile of studies indicates that increased consumption of monounsaturated fatty acids decreases one's overall risk for vessel disease. *Oleic acid*, found in olives and cold-pressed, extra virgin olive oil, appears to prevent hardening of the arteries while lowering the incidence of blood clots, heart attack, and stroke. In fact, the extremely low prevalence of heart disease in southern Europe is largely attributable to the traditional Mediterranean diet, characterized by an exceptionally high concentration of monounsaturated fatty acids.

Polyunsaturated Fatty Acids: The Two-Faced Fats

Polyunsaturated fatty acids contain more than one double bond and are "unsaturated" at two or more points within the carbon chain. Hence, like monounsaturated fatty acids, polyunsaturated fatty acids are kinked and don't like to lie flat. As a result, they also tend to exist as liquids (oils) at room temperature.

The vast majority of polyunsaturated fatty acids consumed in the diet derive from vegetable oils. Vegetable oils that contain the highest concentrations of polyunsaturated fat, including corn oil, safflower oil, sunflower oil, and soybean oil, have long been touted as the healthy alternative to saturated fat. Indeed, early research showed that using these oils instead of butter for cooking could decrease LDL (bad) cholesterol levels. Unfortunately, once again, it appears that the experts jumped to some unsubstantiated conclusions when they began recommending polyunsaturated vegetable oil as a healthy cooking alternative to butter and lard. Recent studies show that although including these vegetable oils in your diet may lower your LDL cholesterol, your overall risk for cardiovascular disease and fatal heart attack will actually *increase*.

How is this possible?

Well, it turns out that LDL cholesterol in and of itself is pretty harmless. However, because polyunsaturated fatty acids contain numerous double bonds, they are much less stable and much more reactive than both saturated fatty acids like butter and monounsaturated fatty acids like olive oil. Just like oxygen in the air can oxidize iron to cause the formation of rust, polyunsaturated fatty acids can oxidize LDL cholesterol. And guess what, it's the *oxidized* form of LDL cholesterol that damages your arteries and induces the formation of artery-narrowing plaques. And the fun doesn't stop there! Polyunsaturated vegetable oils have other deadly talents, including immune system suppression. They are also good for making platelets stickier and increasing the risk for blood clots and stroke.

The more scientists learn about the mechanisms of chronic disease, the more it appears that polyunsaturated vegetable oils exert their dangerous effects by promoting the production of inflammatory compounds in the body. Returning to the concept of homeostasis, inflammation is a giant red flag for disequilibrium and imbalance. In addition to virtually every disease process known to man, inflammation also contributes to weight gain and obesity.

As you know, homeostasis represents an enormously convoluted and precariously balanced venture, accomplished to varying degrees of success thanks to a constant supply of essential matter and energy. The feat of providing every life-sustaining homeostatic process with vital building blocks is an incredibly dynamic juggling act. Homeostasis under the influence of chronic inflammation is like a juggler, well, under the influence. If our tipsy juggler happens to drop a couple of balls, the first thing to go probably won't be the oxygen supply to the brain, but it might be a shipment of amino acids earmarked for muscle toning. Obviously, this example is a far-fetched oversimplification of these exceedingly involved, interdependent, physiological processes. However, it is important to understand that even *subclinical inflammation*, or inflammation that slips under your doctor's radar, causes widespread damage to your health that will ultimately manifest as a myriad of conditions. Everything from heart disease and autoimmune disorders to more aesthetic concerns like poor body composition and wrinkled skin owes its existence to chronic inflammation.

Trans-Fatty Acids: Lethal Lipids

In addition to marbleized beef and polyunsaturated vegetable oils, the turn of the century gave Americans one more reason to die young: *Trans-fatty acids,* which until about a hundred years ago barely existed. Then in 1897 someone got the bright idea to take polyunsaturated vegetable oil and *hydrogenate* it, a process that entails heating the oil to very high temperatures in order to disrupt the double bonds within the carbon chains of the fatty acids. As the double bonds break, the relevant carbon atoms fill their vacated binding sites by grabbing extra hydrogen atoms. Once the double bonds are broken, the kinks in the carbon chains straighten out and, eureka! *Hydrogenated* or *trans* fats are born.

With the absence of double bonded carbons, trans fats are far more stable than their reactive precursors, polyunsaturated vegetable oils. As a result, they enjoy a greatly extended shelf life. From a food manufacturer's perspective, trans-fatty acids have many commercial advantages. They are cheap to make, solid at room temperature, and they don't spoil. Moreover, largely thanks to Senator McGovern's war on fat, until very recently, trans fats were perceived by the general public to be healthier than the saturated fats they replaced.

Commercially, trans fats are used in the production of shortening and margarine, the manufacture of baked goods, and in fast food preparation. They are common ingredients in snack foods, crackers, doughnuts, cakes, microwave popping corn, peanut butter, non-dairy creamers, stick margarine, and many deep-fried fast food items like french fries. If you do not make a conscious effort to avoid them, trans fats will almost surely find a way of sneaking into your diet.

Unfortunately, trans fats are even deadlier than their sinister polyunsaturated precursors. Trans fats significantly decrease HDL (good) cholesterol while raising LDL (bad) cholesterol. Their consumption has been linked to hardening of the arteries of the brain, heart, and kidneys, an elevated incidence of heart attack and stroke, the development of insulin resistance and diabetes, systemic immune suppression, and increased cancer risks. Epidemiological studies suggest that the elimination of trans fats from the American diet could prevent approximately 100,000 premature coronary deaths every year!

Thanks to new legislation, food manufacturers are now required to list the trans fat content of all foods. Needless to say, trans-fatty acids do not play any part in the *Ten Years Thinner* meal plan.

THE LEAN ESSENTIALS:

- Saturated fat, found in all whole food animal protein sources, probably isn't as unhealthy as we have been led to believe.

- Monounsaturated fat, found in high concentrations in olives, avocados, nuts, and seeds, promotes a healthy heart and a firm, youthful physique.

- The polyunsaturated fats that occur in corn, canola, soybean, sunflower, and safflower oil are pro-inflammatory and contribute to heart disease.

- Trans fats are deadly and should be eliminated from the diet altogether.

THE TAKE-HOME MESSAGE ABOUT FAT

When our diet contains the right kinds of fat in the correct proportions, fat is good for us. In fact, the absolute amount of dietary fat we consume is far less important than the relative quantities of specific fatty acids. This tenet applies to both our cardiovascular health and our body composition. But with all the controversy surrounding what constitutes a "healthy" fat intake, how can we determine the best way to eat for both good health and a firm physique?

Luckily, once again, we have the most reliable reality check in the world at our disposal: evolution. If we take a closer look at our Stone Age counterparts, we can learn a lot about healthy fat intake. Research indicates that although the vast majority of the world's hunter-gatherer societies derived about 40 percent of their total caloric intake from dietary fat—a percentage that happens to correspond to the fat content of the average "unhealthy" Western diet—by all evidence, our Stone Age ancestors did not suffer from cardiovascular disease, obesity, or a host of other contemporary ailments. And according to both anthropologists and epidemiologists, the absence of so-called modern diseases among hunter-gatherer societies cannot be wholly attributed to their more active lifestyles.

It turns out that although early humans probably derived about the same percentage of their *total* caloric intake from fat as we do today, the *quality* of their fat intake was very different from ours. For starters, Stone Age humans did not eat commercially prepared baked goods or deep fried fast foods. Hence, their diets were essentially free of the deadly trans-fatty acids that plague our modern menus. Likewise, hunter-gatherers did not have ready access to the polyunsaturated vegetable oils with their ill-boding, pro-inflammatory omega-6 to omega-3 essential fatty acid ratios.

Instead, Stone Age humans obtained their dietary fat primarily from a combination of nuts, which are high in heart-healthy monounsaturated fatty acids, plus the flesh and organs of the animals they hunted and scavenged. Fossil evidence indicates that fish and fowl did not become a significant part of the hunter-gatherer diet until about 25,000 years ago. During the preceding millennia, most hunter-gatherer societies derived the majority of their animal-based foods from wild game.

When researchers compared the meat from modern, grain-fed beef to that of wild game, they discovered some telling differences. For starters, cuts of grain-fed beef contain about *ten times* as much fat as comparable cuts of wild game. And the quality of the fat is very different. Beef fat contains about twice as many saturated fatty acids and less than one-third as many monounsaturated fatty acids. Moreover, the ratio of omega-6 to omega-3 essential fatty acids in grain-fed beef is about twice what is observed in wild game.

By combining anthropological data pertaining to our evolutionary history with what recent studies have revealed about the impact of different fatty acids on human homeostasis, we finally have the information we need to create a meal plan that contains the proper amounts and ratios of specific fatty acids for promoting optimal health, extended longevity, and—of course—a firm, younger-looking physique.

The Canola Conspiracy

By the late eighties, the American Heart Association, the National Institutes of Health, and other U.S. government-funded researchers had squandered millions trying to prove that polyunsaturated vegetable oils were heart healthy and should replace saturated fat whenever possible. But the more we replaced the "unhealthy" saturated fats with "heart-healthy" polyunsaturates like corn and soybean oil, the sicker and fatter we got. Rather than acknowledging that they might have been hasty in their condemnation of saturated fat, government-funded researchers and the processed food industry scrambled to find a new hero to replace the dismal failure of polyunsaturated vegetable oils. That's when Canada came to the rescue with an engineered version of rapeseed known as canola. Unlike "organic" rapeseed which is high in erucic acid, a toxic monounsaturate that causes organ damage, canola seed was genetically manipulated to contain only traces of this poison.

Given the nutrio-political climate of the latter half of the eighties, canola oil seemed like a pretty great invention. It was low in the saturated fat that the American Heart Association doggedly continued to vilify; it was only a fraction as expensive and nearly as high in monounsaturates as olive oil, which was quickly gaining a heart-healthy reputation; and it contained high concentrations of the omega-3 fatty acids that were just making their research debut as benefactors of human immune function. In other words, canola oil was positioned as a politically correct and economically attractive alternative to other vegetable oils. Unfortunately, political correctness rarely correlates with good science or good health.

Canola oil has never undergone vigorous scientific scrutiny. The handful of animal studies that were performed over the last thirty years suggest that it contributes to fibrotic heart lesions, vitamin E deficiency, blood platelet abnormalities, and growth retardation. Processed food and edible-oil industry proponents point to the high concentration of omega-3 fatty acids, arguing that canola oil has cardioprotective properties. What they fail to disclose is that before Canola oil reaches the supermarket aisles, it must first undergo a deodorization process that transforms most of the omega-3s into deadly trans fats. The bottom line: there isn't a study in existence directly linking the consumption of canola oil to decreased cardiac risk in humans. Furthermore, its widespread use since the early nineties has done nothing to derail the trifecta of obesity, diabetes, and heart disease that is spreading across the globe like a medieval plague.

———— ♦♦♦♦♦ ————

"The *Ten Years Thinner* program enabled me to achieve results I never knew were possible, like being able to eat to a full stomach and still, for the first time in my life, have ripped abs!" — DON, 32

"The best thing about the meal plan is you never think about the foods you *can't* have, because you're always thinking about all the foods you *can*! It's such a positive way to approach eating." — JILLIAN, 38

"When I hear the term 'diet,' I think restriction. But this program isn't restrictive. I'm never hungry. Sometimes I actually have trouble finishing the portions. I also never have cravings." — CATHY, 31

———— ♦♦♦♦♦ ————

CHAPTER 4

Carbohydrates Part I:
Friendly Fire for Burning Fat

If you read the opening lines of Chapter 3 and smiled smugly to yourself because you already *knew* that fat was good for your health *and* your lean physique, I think the pages to come will rattle your diet credo to its core.

How can I make such a sweeping assertion? Because if you already *knew* that low-fat eating makes having a firm physique practically impossible, I strongly suspect that you were brainwashed in the nineties by a certain doctor who got rich pushing a remarkably ironic diet—one that simultaneously fosters weight gain and malnutrition. This being the case, I will wager that you suffer from an irrational dread of all things carbohydrate.

OK, take a deep breath. Here comes the shocker: You require lots of carbohydrate in order to achieve and maintain a firm, youthful physique. Carbohydrates play an extremely vital and all too often misunderstood role in sustaining a lean body composition. In fact, of the three macronutrients, carbohydrates have the greatest bearing on the fundamental design of the *Ten Years Thinner* meal plan. A basic understanding of how different carbohydrates impact your overall health and homeostasis is your key to a long, lean existence. As you know, a firm, youthful physique relies on a revved metabolism, which, in turn, relies on a well-oiled homeostasis. The following pages will illustrate why a balanced homeostasis demands the consumption of abundant, healthy carbohydrates.

CARBOHYDRATES AND THE
HORMONES THEY HARNESS

Unfortunately, the anti-carbs craze of the nineties took up where the anti-fat craze of the eighties left off, and with equally catastrophic consequences. The low carbohydrate diets that swept the nineties like social diseases got so popular for a very good reason: initially, they *worked*. People lost weight on them. But within weeks or months, these same people gained all the weight back—plus a bunch more.

Why did this happen?

Before you can fully appreciate the answer to this question, you will need to cleanse your mind of all the carbo-phobic dogma that's been circulating for more than a decade. So, let's start with the basics.

Like protein, carbohydrate contains approximately four calories per gram. The digestion of dietary carbohydrates into their fundamental components begins in the mouth and ends in the small intestine. By the time food reaches your small bowel, a combination of mechanical and enzymatic processes have reduced carbohydrates into single molecules of sugar, otherwise known as *monosaccharides*. Monosaccharides are small enough to be absorbed through the intestinal walls and into the *portal circulation*, which takes them through the liver before they are released into the general circulation. In the liver, all sugars are converted to a specific form of monosaccharide known as *glucose*; hence all sugars in the general circulation exist in the form of glucose.

When you eat a meal that contains carbohydrates, blood glucose levels increase over time. In response to this rise in blood sugar, the pancreas releases the hormone *insulin*, which acts like a glucose chaperone, escorting it out of the general circulation and into tissue cells. The final destination of each glucose molecule is determined by the body's needs. Ideally, insulin directs the first of the arriving glucose to metabolically active tissues, primarily brain, muscle, and red blood cells, where it serves as an immediate fuel source. Insulin then takes as much of the remaining glucose as possible and shepherds it onto liver and muscle tissue where it is stored for future use. To save space, stored glucose molecules are stacked like folding chairs to form a sort of lattice known as *glycogen*. Once all the glycogen storage spaces are full, insulin steers any remaining glucose to lipid deposits (like the ones that make your thighs jiggle) where it gets converted to fat.

THE LEAN ESSENTIALS:

- Digestive processes reduce carbohydrates into single molecules of sugar, known as *monosaccharides,* which are converted to *glucose* before entering the general circulation.

- Glucose that is not used as an immediate fuel source gets stored within liver and muscle tissue in the form of *glycogen.*

Glucose and Insulin: Yin and Yang

If it has been several hours since you ate any carbohydrates, blood glucose levels start to fall and additional fuel must be provided for metabolically active tissues, especially your greedy, glucose-hungry brain. Under these circumstances, the hormone *glucagon* steps in to harness glucose from glycogen stores.

From the standpoint of physiological equilibrium, insulin and glucagon are the yin and yang of blood sugar homeostasis. Both hormones are manufactured by specialized endocrine cells in the pancreas: insulin comes from the *beta cells*, and glucagon comes from the *alpha cells*. Conceptually, you can think of insulin as primarily responsible for clearing glucose out of the bloodstream, and glucagon as primarily responsible for putting glucose back into the bloodstream.

THE LEAN ESSENTIALS:

- The hormone *insulin* is primarily responsible for clearing glucose out of the bloodstream after a meal.

- The hormone *glucagon* is primarily responsible for putting glucose back into the bloodstream after a period of fasting.

HOW LOW-CARB DIETS MAKE YOU FAT

Although the human body is capable of warehousing vast amounts of fat, when it comes to carbohydrate, our bodies have a surprisingly limited storage capacity. The average person can only retain about 75 to 100 grams of liver glycogen, and even the most muscular individual tops off at about 400 grams of muscle glycogen. Whereas liver glycogen represents a viable fuel source for all active tissues, muscles don't share. Once glucose finds its way into your muscle tissue and gets stored as muscle glycogen, it becomes inaccessible to all other tissues and organs. Hence, at any given time, the paltry carbohydrate stores available to your nonmuscle tissue, including your brain, equate to roughly 400 calories worth of liver glycogen, or about the same amount of carbohydrate contained in a slice of pizza.

Limited glycogen storage space is part of the reason that many dietary carbohydrates have a tendency to spill over and wind up stored as fat. Limited glycogen storage is also germane to why low carbohydrate diets don't induce sustainable weight loss. Assuming you don't exercise, the typical low-carbohydrate diet will deplete your glycogen stores in about a day. High levels of physical activity can devour your glycogen stores in just a couple of hours.

The Ketogenic Diet: A Recipe for Disaster

Under conditions of severe carbohydrate restriction and subsequent glycogen depletion, glucagon and other hormones rally to increase the harvest of fat stores for energy. The process of liberating stored fat involves extracting free fatty acids from fat cells and turning them loose in the blood stream. Fatty acids in the systemic circulation are then broken down into smaller, acidic fragments known as *ketone bodies* or simply *ketones,* which can be used as an alternative energy source.

Even with adequate carbohydrate intake and brimming glycogen stores, ketones are normally present in the bloodstream in small amounts. However, when they reach a threshold concentration, ketones threaten to upset the delicate acid-base balance necessary for life-sustaining homeostasis. In response to the increased acidity caused by an accumulation of ketones in the blood stream, the body does all it can to get rid of them. As a result, ketone bodies are dispatched in the urine and you start to pee like there's no tomorrow.

Once ketone bodies begin to appear in your urine, you are said to be in a state of *ketosis,* or simply *ketotic.* Because ketone bodies contain about five calories per gram, in a sense, the ketotic individual is literally peeing away their body fat. However, almost all the weight lost during the initial few days of ketosis has nothing to do with decreased body fat. The first five to seven pounds of weight loss from ketosis is merely a reflection of decreased water retention due to increased urination. Nevertheless, water loss gives dieters a sense of accomplishment because they see their weight plummet by several pounds in a matter of days.

This still sounds pretty great though, doesn't it?

Well, unfortunately, prolonged ketosis has several distinct drawbacks for anyone trying to lose body fat and keep it off. First, ketogenic diets force your body to break down muscle protein in order to liberate amino acids for conversion to glucose. And as you know, muscle loss is absolutely, positively, one hundred percent counterproductive to a lean, toned physique. Every ounce of muscle sacrificed for glucose production incrementally slows your metabolic rate, which ultimately contributes to fat storage.

And second, sustained ketosis turns your fat cells into fat sponges. No matter how much fat and protein you eat, the longer you deprive your body of carbohydrates, the more convinced your body becomes that you are experiencing a famine. In order to keep your brain supplied with what little glucose might become available, your other "less essential" tissues and organs begin to ignore insulin when it comes knocking at their door with a glucose delivery. As a result, blood glucose that is not immediately used as an energy source has a much greater likelihood of winding up stored as fat. In fact, research indicates that ketogenic diets can multiply your affinity for storing fat by *up to tenfold!*

Finally, and perhaps most importantly, ketogenic diets are horribly monotonous! Sure, they might seem great in the beginning. After years of low-fat diet disasters and counting calories to no avail, to the seasoned diet veteran, a meal plan that allows for as much protein and fat as one's heart desires can seem like a dream come true. In fact, if all you want to do is rapidly drop ten or fifteen pounds for, say, a high school reunion, and you don't care about gaining twenty or thirty pounds during the weeks and months following the big event, a ketogenic diet could be exactly what the doctor ordered. Just don't act surprised when you abandon the miracle meal plan and start to pack on the pounds.

To put it simply, a low-carb diet ultimately causes weight gain because it literally primes your body for fat gain. The hormonal modifications caused by a ketogenic diet turn your fat cells into fat sponges while your metabolism takes a nose dive due to muscle loss. Your body becomes thriftier with calories so that you are better able to survive your self-imposed famine. If you think about it from an evolutionary perspective, it makes perfect sense that your body would become more adept at holding onto fat during times of food scarcity. Indeed, the ability to produce ketones as an alternative energy source probably conferred an important survival advantage 30,000 years ago. The fact that famine no longer presents a realistic threat to our survival does not nullify our genetic heritage. Once again, we can ignore our genes, but our genes will not ignore us!

LEAN ESSENTIALS:

- Your body needs adequate amounts of carbohydrate in order to maintain a lean body composition.

- Carbohydrate restriction leads to glycogen depletion, which leads to ketosis.

- Prolonged ketosis can multiply your affinity for storing fat by up to tenfold.

- Prolonged ketosis forces your body to break down muscle protein, which ultimately leads to a sluggish metabolism and fat gain.

FRUITS AND VEGETABLES: THE CLEVEREST OF CARBS

Although avoiding the negative consequences of ketosis is certainly a good reason NOT to eliminate carbohydrates from your diet, it is not the only reason. In fact, it is not even the most compelling reason.

Forty thousand years ago, early humans didn't throw much away. By eating the eyes, brains, marrow, glands, and organs of their prey, our ancestors were able to obtain many vitamins, minerals, enzymes, and other essential nutrients even during times of carbohydrate scarcity. Since humans stopped eating brains and eyeballs and gonads on a regular basis, carbohydrate-rich foods like fruits and vegetables have become our only reliable source for many essential micronutrients including vitamins, minerals, enzymes, and trace elements, not to mention the staggering array of anti-inflammatory antioxidants and phytochemicals that are unique to plant food sources.

Eating between five and nine daily servings of nutrient-rich fruits and vegetables has a tremendously positive impact on our physiological equilibrium. People who consume at least five servings of fresh fruits and vegetables each day enjoy an enormously decreased risk for obesity, diabetes, blood clots, stroke, heart disease, and many forms of cancer. The more fresh fruits and leafy vegetables you eat, the more stable your homeostasis, the better your overall health, and—you guessed it—the younger and leaner your physique.

Furthermore, fruits and vegetables are vital for maintaining bone health, especially if you eat a high protein, muscle-toning diet. Protein metabolism causes an increase in urinary acidity, which has the potential to lead to increased calcium losses. Fruits and vegetables have an *alkalizing* effect that makes urine more basic. Their consumption in adequate quantities counteracts the acidifying effects of protein, protects your kidneys from renal disease and kidney stones, and prevents calcium losses in the urine. The upshot of a diet rich in fruits and vegetables is a skeleton rich in calcium, which is a formidable defense against the bone mineral losses that can accompany aging, especially for postmenopausal women. Moreover, calcium also appears to decrease cancer risks, improve cholesterol profiles, and reduce the risk for life-threatening cardiovascular events like heart attack and stroke. Not to mention that calcium has become an overnight celebrity for enhancing fat loss. Over the past months, study after study has demonstrated a convincing association between increased calcium in the diet and decreased fat retention. So if building a firm, flab-free physique is a priority, calcium should be on your short list of must-have minerals.

Micronutrients and calcium retention are only the tip of the iceberg lettuce! Fruits and leafy vegetables are also high in fiber, which, as you have certainly heard by now, is good for you. All types of fiber have one thing in common: They possess molecular structures that withstand human digestive enzymes. Because fiber is essentially immune to digestion, it never gets broken down and released into the blood stream in the form of glucose. Instead, fiber passes through the gastrointestinal tract largely intact and is eliminated in the stool. Hence, although adequate fiber intake is paramount to stable homeostasis and overall good health, as far as your firm physique is concerned, fiber is calorically vacant: You can eat as much fiber as your heart desires and it will never make you gain an ounce of fat.

THE LEAN ESSENTIALS:

- Fruits and vegetables are the best source of many essential vitamins, minerals, enzymes, trace elements, anti-inflammatory antioxidants, and phytochemicals.

- Fruits and vegetables prevent calcium losses in the urine, which, in turn, combats osteoporosis, cancer, heart disease, and fat gain.

- Fruits and leafy vegetables are the best sources of dietary fiber. Although fiber has zero functional calories, it is vital to a stable homeostasis.

INSOLUBLE FIBER:
FOR HEALTHY GUTS AND YOUNGER SKIN

Insoluble fiber derives from the structural components of plants, mainly the *cellulose* comprising their cell walls, and is present in the bran portion of grains, as well as fruits, vegetables, and legumes. Insoluble fiber adds bulk to stool and softens it. As a result, fecal matter moves easily through the colon, intestinal transit time is decreased, and less pressure is needed to expel stool at the end of the ride. A diet containing ample amounts of insoluble fiber diminishes the risk for a number of serious health concerns including constipation, hemorrhoids, diverticulosis, and colon cancer.

Certain types of insoluble fiber are fermented by the so-called friendly bacteria that normally inhabit the large bowel. Current research indicates that these friendly bacteria are responsible for aiding normal digestive processes, lowering cholesterol, stimulating immune function, preventing malignancy, and ensuring proper macro- and micronutrient absorption. As you know, proper nutrient absorption is pivotal to both stable homeostasis and a firm physique. Unfortunately, not all the microbes that live in our guts are friendly.

The intestines of humans contain 100 trillion viable bacteria, consisting of several hundred individual species. The resident bacteria of the large intestine play a major role in health and nutrition. In the most basic terms, intestinal bacteria can be divided into two groups: species that are harmful to host welfare, and species that are beneficial to host welfare. Harmful or *pathogenic* bacteria produce toxic, inflammatory compounds that contribute to the development of cancer, liver and kidney disease, high blood pressure, heart disease, and wrinkles. A growing number of scientists and health professionals believe that many modern diseases of the GI tract, including irritable bowel syndrome, Crohn's disease, ulcerative colitis, peptic ulcers, food allergies, and premature aging, are linked to colonization of the digestive tract with pathogenic bacterial strains.

Unfortunately, many aspects of modern living can upset the delicate balance of intestinal flora in favor of harmful microbes. Fortunately, something as simple as including enough insoluble fiber in your diet can tip the balance back toward the good guys. The fermentation of dietary fiber by friendly bacteria produces a variety of short-chain fatty acids that are the preferred fuel source for the cells of the large bowel. The health of your colon depends on an adequate supply of these fatty acids, and to a greater extent than you might realize, *your* health depends on the health of your colon. Constipation and colon cancer aside, the cells that line your GI tract form the first line of defense against invading organisms, toxic substances, and a host of other inflammatory agents. The cells of your large bowel are like sentries, guarding your domain. The ability of your sentries to perform their protective duties relies heavily on the symbiotic relationship they maintain with their allies, the friendly bacteria.

And, in turn, the health of your friendly bacteria relies on the quality and quantity of insoluble fiber you choose to include in your diet. Other beneficial products of fermentation include fatty acids that kill pathogenic gut bacteria, fatty acids that are used for fuel by hepatic (liver) and muscle cells, and fatty acids that inhibit the enzyme responsible for cholesterol synthesis in the liver. The production of these fatty acids may contribute to insoluble fiber's cholesterol lowering prowess.

SOLUBLE FIBER: FOR A HEALTHY HEART AND A FIRM PHYSIQUE

Like insoluble fiber, *soluble fiber* derives from vegetation, primarily fleshy fruits, legumes, and vegetables. It consists of substances known as *hydrocolloids*, large molecules that are *hydrophilic*, or "water loving." By virtue of their chemical structures, hydrocolloids can attract and bind up to 200 times their weight in water. In plants, hydrocolloids occur as gums and pectins inside and around the plant's cells where they facilitate fluid retention, enabling the plant to stay hydrated. When we eat plant matter, or take soluble fiber as a supplement, the hydrocolloids expand and thicken to form an amorphous gel as they pass through the gastrointestinal tract. Soluble fiber decreases the rate of gastric emptying and contributes to a feeling of fullness that may help prevent overeating, which is more good news for your firm physique.

Research indicates that soluble fiber also lowers serum cholesterol levels. This is probably related to soluble fiber's ability to inhibit the absorption of both dietary cholesterol and bile from the GI tract. Bile, which is necessary for normal fat digestion, is manufactured by the liver from cholesterol substrates, and then sent to the gallbladder where it is concentrated and stored. When dietary fat reaches the stomach, it causes the release of the hormone *cholecystokinin*, which, as we touched on in Chapter 3, informs the brain that we are getting full. Cholecystokinin also signals the gallbladder to secrete bile into the small bowel to emulsify fatty acids for increased digestibility.

In the normal course of bile circulation, bile that has been sent to the small bowel is resorbed and recycled. However, soluble fiber acts like a bile and cholesterol sponge, soaking up both dietary cholesterol and old, worn-out bile that may contribute to the formation of gallstones, and delivering them straight to the toilet. Hence, soluble fiber obliges the liver to synthesize fresh, new bile from a diminished supply of incoming cholesterol substrates. This explains how a diet that is high in soluble fiber both prevents gallstones and lowers cholesterol.

Although scientists still have a great deal to learn about the many health-promoting attributes of soluble fiber, its greatest virtue could very well prove to be its ability to prevent a flabby physique and heart disease by functionally lowering the *glycemic index* of ingested foods. (I will elaborate further on the concept of glycemic index and glycemic load in Chapter 5.)

THE LEAN ESSENTIALS:

- Fiber prevents gallstones, constipation, hemorrhoids, diverticulosis, colon cancer, heart disease, and obesity.

- *Insoluble fiber* tips the balance in favor of "friendly" gut bacteria, which are paramount to a healthy GI tract, proper nutrient absorption, and younger-looking skin.

- *Soluble fiber* contributes to a feeling of fullness and functionally lowers the glycemic index of your meal. Both attributes help prevent insulin resistance, heart disease, and a flabby physique.

———— ✦✦✦✦✦ ————

"I was afraid I'd feel tired if I cut out
sugar and starchy carbohydrates, but by the end of
the first week, I felt super energetic and
I didn't miss the sugar at all." — DARLENE, 43

"I used to crave cookies and coffee every day at four o'clock,
and junk food in the evenings. Once I started the program,
I was so focused on all the things I *could* eat, I literally
stopped thinking about all the things I *couldn't.*
I haven't had a cookie craving like that since
my second day on the program." — JILLIAN, 38

"I used to be a carbo junkie. My biggest concern
when I started *Ten Years Thinner* was that I wouldn't be
able to give up the bad carbs. I love pasta; I love bread;
I love french Fries. But my cravings were completely
eliminated within the first few days. *Gone.* And I
don't miss those foods. The program literally changed
what I have an appetite for." — MATT, 38

———— ✦✦✦✦✦ ————

CHAPTER 5

Carbohydrates Part II: Glycemic Response and the Bane of the Grain

The *glycemic index* was first developed in 1981 by a team of scientists lead by Dr. David Jenkins, a professor of nutrition at the University of Toronto. The glycemic index of a food is a scaled, numeric representation of the insulin response elicited by that particular food item. As you know from Chapter 4, insulin, which is produced and secreted by the pancreas, is the hormone responsible for getting glucose out of the bloodstream.

In essence, the end product of all edible carbohydrate digestion is a variable ratio of three different monosaccharides, each with its own unique molecular structure. *Glucose* is the only monosaccharide that our tissues can utilize directly. In order for *fructose* (found mainly in fruit) and *galactose* (found mainly in dairy products) to become available fuel sources, they must first be converted to glucose within the liver. As they pass through the liver, the process of converting nonglucose monosaccharides into glucose slows their release into the general circulation. As a result, carbohydrate foods that contain mainly nonglucose monosaccharides (like fruits, vegetables, and dairy products) tend to enter the bloodstream more gradually than carbohydrate foods that break down mostly into glucose (like bread, pasta, cereal, corn, rice, and potatoes).

The rapidity with which a given food item is delivered into the bloodstream in the form of glucose determines the magnitude of its insulin response. Foods that find their way into the bloodstream gradually produce minimum insulin responses and are said to have *low glycemic indices*. Carbs with the lowest glycemic indices include fruits, leafy vegetables, legumes, and yams. Conversely, foods that flood the general circulation with glucose induce a surge of insulin, often referred to as an *insulin spike*. These foods are said to have *high glycemic indices* and include processed and/or refined cereal grains, regular soda, alcoholic beverages, and seemingly more innocuous carbohydrate sources like fruit juice, potatoes, and corn.

THE LEAN ESSENTIALS:

- Carbohydrate foods that find their way into the bloodstream gradually (fruits, leafy vegetables, legumes, and yams) produce minimal insulin responses and are said to have low glycemic indices.

- Carbohydrate foods that flood the general circulation with glucose induce a surge of insulin. These foods, which include processed and/or refined cereal grains (i.e., bread products, pasta, and white rice), regular soda, alcoholic beverages, fruit juice, potatoes, and corn, are said to have high glycemic indices.

HOW HIGH GLYCEMIC FOODS MAKE YOU FAT AND OLD

The higher the glycemic index of a food, the greater the insulin response it will elicit. When consumed by themselves, foods with high glycemic indices literally flood your systemic circulation with glucose. The pancreas, sensing a sharp rise in blood glucose, leaps into action to subvert the threat of high blood sugar, otherwise known as *hyperglycemia*. High blood sugar is exceedingly unhealthy for your body and your pancreas knows it. Over time, repeated bouts of hyperglycemia cause irreversible damage to nerves, blood vessels, and organs. Poorly controlled blood sugar is the primary reason that diabetics are at a substantially increased risk for kidney disease, heart attack, blindness, and amputation.

Unfortunately, when the pancreas gets wind of an extremely rapid rise in blood glucose, it tends to overcompensate with an insulin spike. As a result, *too much* glucose is cleared *too rapidly* from your bloodstream. This creates a situation of low blood sugar, or *hypoglycemia*. Your greedy, glucose-hungry brain doesn't put up with hypoglycemia. As you might recall from Chapter 1, brain cells or *neurons* are the only cells in the human body that are even more metabolically active than muscle cells. Your brain requires a constant energy supply and glucose is the neurons' fuel of choice. Lucky for your gray matter, your brain is ideally situated to get what it wants because it controls your behavior.

When a dive in blood sugar makes us irritable, unfocused, and hungry (even though we just devoured an entire box of donut holes), our brain leaps into action and we start thinking how delicious another box of donut holes would taste right now! In fact, the sugar cravings induced by hypoglycemia send many people running to the cupboards or the candy machine or the corner store for more of the same high glycemic index foods that caused the problem in the first place. High glycemic index foods can easily create a vicious cycle of carbohydrate bingeing that leads to a rapid rise in blood sugar which, in turn, leads to an insulin spike and hypoglycemia—which, of course, leads right back to carbohydrate bingeing.

What happens to all the glucose once it's cleared from the circulation? Some of it is stored as glycogen in our liver and muscle tissue. But when that limited storage space becomes full, any glucose that doesn't get crammed into a glycogen lattice spills over and winds up stored as fat. Although excess body fat is unsightly (and definitely counterproductive to building a firm physique), there are far more sinister ramifications of a diet that includes too many high glycemic index carbohydrates.

You see, every time your pancreas senses a rapid rise in blood glucose it goes on red alert and spews out an insulin spike. After responding to so many red alerts, other tissues in the body begin to think that the pancreas is just crying wolf. These tissues literally become desensitized to insulin and lock their doors to glucose entry. Once insulin resistance sets in, it takes an even *bigger* insulin spike to persuade cells to open their doors to glucose. To make matters worse, all those red alerts start to take a toll on the pancreatic beta cells that are responsible for manufacturing the insulin in the first place. The unremitting demands of repeated insulin spikes drain the poor little beta cells of their will to go on. Eventually, some of the overworked beta cells give up and stop making insulin altogether. Of course, the more they burn out, the harder the remaining beta cells have to work to continue producing enough insulin to generate bigger and bigger spikes. Eventually, all the beta cells succumb to exhaustion and the pancreas closes shop to insulin production.

And voila! You've got yourself a case of Type II diabetes mellitus. Congratulations! Now you can look forward to a (shortened) lifetime of glucose monitoring, medication, irreversible organ damage, and gradual, systemic deterioration. All because of a nasty, high-glycemic-index carb habit.

Before developing full-blown diabetes or heart disease, there is a more or less asymptomatic period that can last for several years, during which tissues become increasingly insulin resistant. This phase, alternately referred to as "prediabetes," "metabolic syndrome," or "Syndrome X," is on the rise among all segments of the American population, even teens and tweens. An estimated 50 million people, or roughly one-quarter of all adults in the United states, are currently in the process of building a resistance to insulin. Tragically, because most of the diagnostic criteria for Metabolic Syndrome are considered borderline health risks, many individuals who fit the profile fly under the radar, their condition undetected by their health-care providers until it's too late.

If ignorance is bliss, undiagnosed insulin resistance promises to be a brief bliss. In a sense, Metabolic Syndrome is the last stop on the *Heart Attack Express* before the end of the line. Individuals who don't bother changing trains and cleaning up their eating habits during the prediabetic phase might not enjoy the remainder of their journey very much. Insulin resistance is your last stop before, well, your *last* stop!

Just in case the specter of diabetes isn't enough to make you question your morning bowl of Krispy Sugar Clumps with a side of toast and jam, I've got more bad news about high glycemic index carbohydrates. In addition to conferring a predisposition for diabetes, heart disease, obesity, blindness, and wrinkles, high-glycemic-index carbs wreak havoc on stable homeostasis via countless intersecting processes that scientists are only beginning to unravel.

For example, the quantity of high glycemic index carbohydrates contained in your diet is the single greatest dietary predictor for diminished HDL (good) cholesterol. Moreover, blood glucose reacts with LDL (bad) cholesterol and oxidizes it. (If you recall from Chapter 3, only the oxidized form of LDL cholesterol causes vessel damage.) In fact, it is probably the propensity for blood glucose to react with and oxidize blood-borne substances that makes hyperglycemia so dangerous and makes glucose such a potent inflammatory agent. As you know, chronic, widespread inflammation damages homeostasis, contributing to a host of illnesses from cancer to heart disease, as well as premature aging and weight gain.

INSULIN'S DIRTY LITTLE SECRET

Perhaps not surprisingly, it turns out that it's not just excess blood glucose that promotes inflammation and chronic disease. The *excess insulin* resulting from the *excess blood glucose* is also extremely pro-inflammatory, pro-aging, and pro-chronic disease. Researchers believe that excess insulin can signal cancer cells to multiply (and excess blood glucose supplies them with the fuel they need to do so). In addition, excess insulin leads to insulin resistance, and insulin-resistant tissues are more likely to mount inappropriate inflammatory responses that encourage chronic disease. For example, insulin-resistant neurons are more likely to display the cellular changes consistent with Alzheimer's disease. In fact, people suffering from chronic inflammatory conditions like asthma, acne, multiple sclerosis, and rheumatoid arthritis can often improve (and sometimes even eliminate) their symptoms by cutting high glycemic index carbohydrates out of their diet.

More apropos of your firm physique, the excess insulin triggered by excess blood glucose inhibits your ability to utilize stored fat as an energy source. In addition, increased body fat causes the increased production of pro-inflammatory compounds, which, in turn, lead to even more weight gain. In a nutshell, the consumption of high glycemic index carbohydrates leads to excess insulin release. Excess insulin first *makes* you fat, and then it *keeps* you fat.

THE LEAN ESSENTIALS:

- Over time, a diet that includes large quantities of high glycemic index carbohydrates promotes insulin resistance.

- Insulin resistance contributes to chronically elevated insulin levels and blood glucose, both of which foster widespread inflammation, premature aging, chronic disease, and weight gain.

- Insulin resistance makes you fat and keeps you fat.

DISARMING DANGEROUS CARBS

Does all of this mean that in order to enjoy a full, healthy life and a firm, fab physique you must give up all breads, pasta, desserts, and alcohol forever? No. But it does mean you will probably need to cut back on high glycemic index carbohydrate intake and adopt strategies for rendering the remaining high glycemic index carbs in your diet as harmless as possible. It's actually quite simple to disarm a high glycemic index carbohydrate by *functionally* lowering its glycemic index, hence decreasing its insulin response. How do you take the "high" out of high glycemic index?

Well, sometimes you don't need to. When researchers conduct studies to determine the glycemic index of different carbohydrates, they use a standard 50-gram serving (about 200 calories worth) of the food they are indexing. Based on these testing methods, some foods that do not induce an insulin spike generated surprisingly high glycemic indices. For example, watermelon rings in at a whopping 72 out of a possible 100 on the glucose scale, putting it in the same range as table sugar, white bread, and corn flakes. However, in order to consume 200 calories worth of watermelon quickly enough to induce a rapid rise in blood glucose, you'd have to wolf down over four pounds in one short sitting.

Which brings me to a general rule of thumb for fruits and vegetables: Although they are carbohydrate food sources, you can eat as many fruits and leafy vegetables as your heart desires and they will never make you fat, nor will they promote insulin resistance. In fact, fresh fruit and raw vegetables are so packed with vitamins, minerals, antioxidants, phytochemicals, and fiber, they represent your single most powerful weapon *against* getting fat and developing chronic disease. An ample intake of fresh fruit and vegetables is one of the cornerstones to the *Ten Years Thinner* meal plan.

Aside from the total carbohydrate content and glycemic index of the various food items on your plate, several other factors influence the insulin response of a meal.

First, the greater the meal's fiber content, the slower the food will be digested and absorbed, and the more gradually glucose will reach the general circulation. A high fiber meal generates only a fraction of the insulin response induced by the identical meal minus the fiber. In addition, as you know from Chapter 4, soluble fiber slows gastric emptying and creates a sense of fullness that helps to prevent overeating.

Second, the more fat the meal contains, the slower it will be absorbed into the portal circulation and the more gradually its glucose load will be delivered into the bloodstream. This explains, in part, why the fat-free eighties actually wound up making us fatter. Remember all those fat-free snacks that erupted onto the shelves of your grocery store during the fat-free eighties? Guess what the fat-free snack manufacturers replaced the fat with? High-glycemic-index *sugar*! Brainwashed by all the fat-phobic propaganda propagated by the McGovern committee, the NIH, and the American Heart Association, the eighties consumer was duped into thinking that fat-free snacks and desserts were a viable means to lose body fat. But fat-free snacks didn't help anyone lose body fat. They did accomplish something, though: Fat-free snacks popularized vicious-cycle bingeing and hypoglycemia until the behavior pattern evolved into the hip, alternative lifestyle still practiced by many today.

And last but not least, the naturally occurring acids found in certain foods like citrus fruit, tomatoes, and yogurt can significantly decrease the insulin response to a meal. Along with fat and fiber, natural acids decrease the rate of gastric emptying, digestion, the absorption of monosaccharides, and ultimately, the delivery of glucose into the general circulation. Although citrus fruits and yogurt work to acidify stomach contents, they paradoxically wind up making urine more basic. Hence, including these foods with your meal will not cause calcium wasting in the urine.

THE LEAN ESSENTIALS:

- Between their low glycemic loads and high vitamin, mineral, antioxidant, phytochemical, and fiber content, fruits and vegetables represent our most powerful weapon against disease, aging, and a flabby physique.

- The glycemic index of carbohydrates can be functionally lowered by increasing the fiber content, fat content, and/or acidity of the meal.

A WORD ON HEALTHY CARB CONSUMPTION

Hopefully you're starting to get a sense of how important it is to include adequate amounts of the *right types* of carbohydrates in your diet. Fresh fruits and leafy vegetables are the cornerstone of healthy carb consumption. Because of their high fiber and moisture content, fruits and vegetables are a filling, delicious, low-calorie way to help ensure an adequate intake of essential vitamins, minerals, antioxidants, and phytochemicals. In addition, the alkalinizing effect fresh fruits and vegetables have on our urine makes them one of the most powerful weapons in our arsenal against osteoporosis. Moreover, between their anti-inflammatory qualities, their low glycemic indices, and their soluble fiber content, fresh fruits and vegetables are perhaps our best protection against the development of insulin resistance, obesity, diabetes, heart disease, and all the negative health sequelae commonly associated with Metabolic Syndrome. Substituting fresh fruits and leafy vegetables for high glycemic index carbohydrates is like donning armor against disease, aging, and weight gain.

Enough about fruits and vegetables. What about everything else? What about grains? We've seen that refined and processed grain products like white flour and white rice have high glycemic indices, but not all grains are refined, and some, like unprocessed oats, have relatively low glycemic indices. What about those? It's time to turn our attention back to the ultimate reality check, *evolution*.

THE BANE OF THE GRAIN

Until 10,000 years ago—a mere blink of an eye compared to our genetic life span—the environment that dictated our genetic makeup did not include grains. Unlike the birds, rodents, and grazers that are able to consume grains without suffering negative effects, our ancestors, the primates, did not evolve in the savanna. We spent the first several million years of our evolutionary history in tropical forests eating an entirely different class of plant. As a result, we were never physiologically equipped to digest, absorb, and assimilate grains in a way that promotes well-balanced homeostasis and a strong, healthy body.

Even Prey Fights Back!

As with all other life forms on earth, plant species endure thanks to random adaptations that happen to provide a survival advantage. Natural selection is a compassionless force. Plants that are lucky enough to evolve favorable adaptations enjoy increased reproductive opportunities, while less suited species vanish into the obscurity of extinction. Obviously, species that are best equipped to defend themselves against predators have a better shot at reproducing. As you might expect, over the millions of years that comprised their genetic history, cereal grains evolved a number of elaborate defense strategies to protect themselves against consumption by herbivores.

For example, virtually every cereal grain produces pro-inflammatory *antinutrients*, small proteins that disrupt normal human physiology. A variety of antinutrients common to wheat, oats, barley, corn, and rice have been linked to organ damage, hypersensitivity reactions, and autoimmune disorders. *Lectins*, sticky substances that can bind to many tissues, are the best known class of antinutrients. When lectins adhere to intestinal tissues, they damage cells and interfere with the normal digestion and absorption of nutrients.

Even more alarming, the most widely studied lectin, *wheat germ agglutinin* (WGA), has been definitively identified as the causative agent in at least two autoimmune disorders, *celiac disease*, a serious absorptive disorder, and *dermatitis herpetiformis*, a chronic skin condition characterized by a scaly, itchy rash that can appear almost anywhere on the body including the face.

AUTOIMMUNE DISEASE AND
THE GRAIN FACTOR

Why do autoimmune disorders occur in some people and not in others? Nobody knows for sure. Scientists believe that their genesis is the product of a hereditary predisposition (a genetic component) combined with an environmental stimulus (possibly dietary or microbial). It also seems clear that the more environmental stressors there are challenging your immune system at any given time, the greater your overall inflammatory status, and the lower your threshold for experiencing an autoimmune reaction.

An autoimmune disorder begins when white blood cells that patrol your blood and tissues in search of foreign protein invaders, like bacteria, viruses, and parasites, misidentify "self" tissues as the enemy. When this occurs, white blood cells call in reinforcements and organize an inflammatory response designed to attack and destroy. Unfortunately, in the case of an autoimmune response, the attack is directed at the self, resulting in the destruction of self tissue. Foreign proteins that resemble proteins found in normal human tissue can trick your immune system into mounting a response against your own tissue.

Because many cereal grain antinutrients are resistant to *human proteases* (the enzymes responsible for protein digestion), antinutrients can remain intact as they pass through the digestive tract. Once lectins reach the small bowel, they bind to cells that line the intestines and increase gut permeability. This might explain how lectins like WGA penetrate our GI tract to gain access to our bloodstream. Once they're in, lectins and other antinutrients become ideal candidates for instigating autoimmune reactions.

In fact, a preponderance of evidence has implicated cereal grain antinutrients in the genesis of numerous different autoimmune disorders. WGA is believed to be the causative agent in many cases of insulin-dependent (type 1 or juvenile) diabetes mellitus, rheumatoid arthritis, multiple sclerosis, Sjogren's Syndrome, IgA nephritis, and canker sores. In patients suffering from celiac disease, cereal grains are suspected to contribute to schizophrenia, autism, epilepsy, and a number of crippling neuromuscular conditions.

No More Bread? Say It Ain't So!

Obviously, grains can be consumed in moderate quantities by most people without causing any overt signs of disease. Unfortunately, if you think about it, *covert* disease and widespread, low-grade, chronic inflammation is what usually does us in! By the time the symptoms of chronic illnesses like diabetes, autoimmune disorders, cancer, and heart disease manifest, the damage has already been done and it is often too late to reverse the degenerative changes that will impact the quality of the remainder of our lives.

We did not evolve eating grains. For eons the natural selection that shaped our genetic makeup was largely remote from the influence of cereal grains. As a result, human physiology is ill equipped to harness them as a significant energy source. Nevertheless, foods made from grain are a ubiquitous part of our diet and our culture. It is extremely difficult, remarkably inconvenient, and (unless you suffer from a medical condition related to grain consumption) probably a tad excessive to eliminate them entirely from your diet. However, for the sake of your smooth skin and firm physique, you might be surprised by how simple it is to substantially *limit* your grain intake and not really miss it much at all.

———— ❭❭❭❭❭ ————

"My energy levels are HUGE on this program.
I was really surprised how quickly they improved." — DARLENE, 43

"I sleep so well now that I always have lots of energy.
I don't even bother setting my alarm anymore." — ALEX, 35

"I have way more energy!" — LAURIE, 43

———— ❬❬❬❬❬ ————

CHAPTER 6

Micronutrients that Keep You Lean and Wrinkle-Free

Theoretically speaking, a Stone Age diet would supply all essential nutrients in the proper amounts and ratios for a healthy, steadfast homeostasis. If you could eat like humans ate 10,000 years ago, you would not need to take any nutritional supplements. Unfortunately, duplicating a prehistoric diet is a tall order in today's world. Fundamental changes to our food supply have made it very difficult to consume adequate quantities of certain nutrients solely from whole food sources.

For example, agricultural "advances" now produce larger crops at faster rates. Unfortunately, this artificially accelerated growth precludes the optimal assimilation of nutrients by the plant. As a result, the quantities of vitamins and minerals in fruits and vegetables have significantly declined over the past 20 years. To make matters worse, the regular consumption of nutrient-poor cereal grains displaces the nutrient-rich fruits and vegetables that we evolved eating. As you know from previous chapters, these same cereal grains also increase the essential fatty acid imbalance caused by the consumption of modern livestock versus wild game.

The good news is, by following the guidelines of the *Ten Years Thinner* meal plan, your diet will be rich in antioxidants, as well as essential vitamins and minerals. However, unless you plan to permanently eliminate all cereal grains from your diet and eat only organically grown fruits and vegetables, I do recommend supplementing with a quality multivitamin every day.

But what about the pro-inflammatory imbalance of essential fatty acids in our modern diet? Lamentably, it is now virtually impossible to consume a healthy ratio of omega-3 to omega-6 EFAs without supplementation.

WHY NOT JUST EAT FISH?

For years, the strong association between increased coldwater fish consumption and a decreased risk for heart disease compelled me to recommend eating two to three fish meals per week. Then many ominous studies highlighting the dangers of the toxic levels of heavy metals and polychlorinated biphenyls (PCBs) in seafood forced me to withdraw this recommendation. Despite all the emerging research that supported fish oil supplementation as the miraculous, anti-inflammatory solution to our hazardously pro-inflammatory environment, I was reluctant to recommend taking fish oil until an independent laboratory published a long list of fish oil suppliers whose products had tested negative for both mercury and PCBs. Since then, I have closely followed the growing stockpile of research pertaining to fish oil supplementation and I now fervently promote it as the cornerstone to balanced homeostasis, lean body composition, and young, elastic skin.

Omega-3's: the Fountain of Youth in a Gel Cap

Fish oil's numerous health benefits have been attributed to its extremely high overall concentration of *omega-3 essential fatty acids.* In contrast to the pro-inflammatory omega-6 fatty acids that are rampant in polyunsaturated vegetable oils and grain-based foods, the omega-3 polyunsaturated fatty acids from coldwater fish actually *reduce* the body's production of inflammatory compounds. The flesh of coldwater fish contains large quantities of *eicosapentaenoic acid* (EPA) and *docosahexaenoic acid* (DHA), omega-3 essential fatty acids that have proven to be instrumental in both disease prevention and weight loss. Not surprisingly, compared to our modern eating habits, the hunter-gatherer diet of early humans was plentiful in these omega-3 essential fatty acids. All available research indicates that humans evolved eating a diet that included an omega-3 to omega-6 essential fatty acid ratio that was about *five times* as high as the remarkably pro-inflammatory Western diet consumed by the average unhealthy American. It would take hundreds of pages to detail the litany of health benefits conferred by fish oil supplementation. Below, I have summarized the highlights.

Fish Oil Wards off Chronic Disease

Omega-3 essential fatty acids don't just lower bad cholesterol, they also raise good cholesterol while decreasing the risk of heart disease and heart attack. Fish oil supplementation has also been credited with boosting immune function, lowering blood pressure, and reducing your risk for vessel disease, stroke, obesity, autoimmune disease, and diabetes. In addition, this Lamborghini of lipids is proving to be an important adjunct in the prevention and treatment of many autoimmune disorders ranging from rheumatoid arthritis to inflammatory bowel disease, eczema, asthma, and multiple sclerosis. As if all this wasn't enough to make you want to guzzle the stuff by the gallon, emerging research shows a strong correlation between the increased consumption of dietary fish oil and a decreased risk for all five of the most prevalent forms of cancer—breast, lung, colon, prostate, and skin. Fish oil supplementation has also been experimentally shown to help combat existing malignancy.

Fish Oil Makes You Smart and Keeps You Sane

Omega-3 EFAs are found in extremely high concentrations in your brain and retina. In children, increased consumption of DHA has been linked to improved vision and mental development. Likewise, in elderly populations, fish and fish oil consumption is associated with a decreased risk of dementia, Alzheimer's disease, and macular degeneration. In fact, the consumption of fish and fish oil appears to decrease the incidence of psychosis, depression, and stress-induced rage. One study went so far as to predict that a diet containing adequate amounts of omega–3 EFAs could prevent most psychotic episodes and render neurodegenerative disorders, such as Alzheimer's and dementia, largely avoidable.

Fish Oil Makes You Skinny

The increased consumption of fish and fish oil appears to have numerous beneficial effects on metabolism and weight loss. By reducing the insulin response to high glycemic carbohydrates, fish oil demonstrates a protective effect against both the development of insulin resistance and its progression to type 2 diabetes. In addition, emerging research indicates that omega–3 EFAs triple the expression of specific genes related to intracellular fat burning. What does this mean for your firm physique? In a nutshell, supplementation with fish oil increases weight loss, decreases fat retention (especially in the abdominal area), and encourages the use of stored fat as a fuel source. Fish oil also appears to decrease muscle breakdown, which, as you know, contributes to a revved metabolism and accelerated weight loss.

Fish Oil Keeps You Looking and Feeling Younger

You read right! In human skin, fish oil can help prevent both *photoaging*, caused by exposure to ultraviolet (UV) light, as well as the cosmetic signs of aging resulting from the passage of time. Topically applied fish oil has actually been shown to increase collagen and elastic fiber production in human skin. But the anti-aging effects of omega-3's aren't just skin deep! Fish oil supplementation also appears to decrease the degradation and inflammation associated with osteoarthritis, the most common cause of joint pain, stiffness, and loss of mobility associated with aging.

THE LEAN ESSENTIALS:

- Modern eating habits and changes to our food supply have made it nearly impossible to ingest adequate amounts of the omega–3 essential fatty acids found in fish oil.

- Fish oil has a protective effect against cancer, autoimmune disorders, blindness, dementia, psychosis, heart disease, diabetes, arthritis, weight gain, and the cosmetic signs of aging.

- Fish oil supplementation is paramount to balanced homeostasis, lean body composition, and young, elastic skin. (See Appendices A and B for specific dose recommendations.)

CALCIUM: THE MODERN PARADOX

Everyone knows that calcium is good for your bones. According to the experts, people who eat a Western diet are highly unlikely to consume enough calcium solely from whole food sources. As predicted by these same experts, low bone mineral density—the precursor to osteoporosis—is rampant among not just our aging population, but our population in general. Furthermore, emerging research seems to suggest that adequate calcium intake plays an important role in both fat burning and weight management, and that supplementation may reduce your risk for heart attack, stroke, and certain forms of cancer. In light of all these wonderful attributes, supplementing with calcium seems like a no-brainer.

But just wait one minute, Dr. Dents!—Do I hear a bullfrog? For every study that supports increased dairy and calcium intake for better health, there is another study that seems to refute the first. So what's going on? Well, as you know from Chapter 1, every single component of life-sustaining homeostasis is inextricably linked to every other. It stands to reason that calcium affects a myriad of physiological processes, and that its healthful consumption relies on countless factors. Perhaps now would be a good time to consult the great reality check.

Why Cavemen Had Strong Bones

According to anthropologists, our Stone Age ancestors consumed only a fraction of the currently recommended amounts of calcium. Nevertheless, the fossil record indicates that these prehistoric humans had well-mineralized, fracture-resistant bones. Are there differences between our modern lifestyle and that of our Stone Age counterparts that might explain this discrepancy? Indeed there are!

For starters, exercise increases bone strength and, according to anthropologists, Paleolithic man was far more physically active than we are today. Plus, although early humans subsisted on a diet that would be considered calcium deficient by today's standards, they consumed large quantities of vegetation. As you might recall from Chapter 4, fruits and vegetables decrease the acidity of urine which, in turn, increases calcium retention. But acid-base balance is just one of many factors that influence calcium metabolism. For example, every grain of salt you eat causes your body to excrete some calcium. And wouldn't you know it, *Stone Age man didn't salt his food!* Not surprisingly, a number of studies have demonstrated an undeniable correlation between sodium intake, calcium losses, and decreases in bone density.

In addition to the widespread use of salt, the advent of civilization was also responsible for the domestication of livestock and the introduction of dairy foods. One might think that the addition of such notoriously rich sources of calcium as milk and cheese might offset the deleterious effects of salt. Unfortunately, as with all matters of homeostasis, it's not quite that simple.

The Irony

You see, stable homeostasis and optimal calcium utilization require a balanced intake of calcium relative to magnesium. And while our Stone Age ancestors enjoyed a diet that was rife with magnesium-rich fruits and vegetables, we have adopted a meal plan based on magnesium-poor cereal grains. Moreover, dairy foods boast a calcium to magnesium ratio that is roughly *twelve times* higher than what we evolved eating.

Between dairy foods and grains, the typical Western diet boasts a calcium to magnesium ratio that is three to four times greater than that of our robust Stone Age ancestors. The hormonal modifications brought about by this imbalance not only contribute to bone loss and osteoporosis, but also appear to play a prominent role in the development and progression of type 2 diabetes, hypertension, heart disease, and heart attack. In fact, thanks to their sinister mineral ratios, one of the biggest contributing factors to the development of both osteoporosis and heart disease may be the very same calcium-rich dairy products and whole grains that the so-called experts have been encouraging us to eat for the *prevention* of these conditions.

It is highly unlikely that the grain and dairy industries are about to advertise this fact. Nevertheless, a growing number of studies comparing calcium and magnesium intake for the prevention of osteoporosis, diabetes, hypertension, and heart disease have yielded results that seem to indicate that magnesium supplementation may be even more important than calcium supplementation.

What's a Modern Human to Do?

Well, unless you spend the better part of your existence consuming an extremely low sodium diet, I recommend calcium supplementation. However, calcium supplementation, and/or the regular consumption of dairy products, should always be accompanied by magnesium supplementation.

THE LEAN ESSENTIALS:

- Salt in food leads to calcium losses that contribute to fragile bones, osteoporosis, weight gain, hypertension, heart disease, and heart attack.

- For proper calcium utilization, there must be a balanced intake of magnesium.

- Because the Western diet contains roughly three to four times the healthy ratio of calcium to magnesium, calcium supplementation should always be accompanied by magnesium supplementation. (See Appendices A and B for specific dose recommendations.)

For research updates on fish oil, magnesium, and other nutritional supplements, and for more information on choosing reputable brands, please visit the *Ten Years Thinner* Web site at www.tenyearsthinner.com.

———— ✦✦✦✦✦ ————

"Even though I have a regular exercise regime incorporating dance and weights, I still use Chris's regimen in between two to three times a week. It is particularly effective in helping me stay toned when I travel (which is quite a bit as a food and wine publicist) and I don't need a gym or special equipment to do it." — SERRY OSMENA, 44 (FORMER INTERNATIONAL AEROBIC CHAMPION)

"The *Ten Years Thinner* workout gave me the definition in my arms, abs, and legs that I don't get from cardio. I also love how my hamstrings and glutes look fuller and firmer." — KIM, 39

"I've always done lots of long cardio and still struggled with how I looked. Thanks to *Ten Years Thinner*, I spend about one-third of the time I used to spend exercising, and I'm in the best shape of my life." — DARLENE, 43

"I look and feel better now on *Ten Years Thinner* than I did fifteen years ago when I used to spend a lot more time exercising." — JILLIAN, 38

———— ✦✦✦✦✦ ————

CHAPTER 7

Exercise:
Why Smart Is
Better than Long

So far, you've been treated to a crash course in good nutrition with almost no mention of how to exercise your soon-to-be spectacular physique. There is a reason I waited this long to bring up exercise: Before addressing such a sensitive issue, I wanted to first earn your trust. Hopefully, by this point in my narrative, I've convinced you that I know what I'm talking about.

For many, exercise is an intimidating topic mired with guilty associations. After all, even the most sedentary person has at some point resolved to become more active. Millions of Americans squander millions of dollars every year on running shoes that never wear out, gym memberships that usually do, and pieces of exercise equipment that wind up in our garages collecting dust. It is a well-documented fact that despite our best intentions and repeated attempts to get fit and stay that way, most people give up within a few months of starting a new exercise program.

Bodacious body aside, we are well aware that physical activity lowers cardiac and cancer risks while promoting bone health, gastrointestinal health, and even mental health. How can anybody *not* know just how swell exercise is when the media is constantly bombarding us with glittery factoids *proving* that active individuals have more energy, experience better sleep, are less prone to anxiety, depression, and illness, and enjoy higher self-esteem than the rest of us? (Who wouldn't have higher self-esteem with that litany of superior attributes!) Many of the estimated three out of four adults who do not get the minimal amounts of exercise necessary for basic good health cannot help but harbor feelings of shame about their inadequate activity levels.

It's not your fault!

The reason that we cannot stick to an exercise program is *not* because we lack the willpower, or the dedication, or even the time. The reason we cannot stick to an exercise program is because ***most exercise programs do not work***. Just like low-fat and low-carb diets don't work, the vast majority of exercise routines that are compact enough to fit into our busy schedules are inefficient for promoting appreciable changes in body composition or improvements in health. Not only that, most exercise programs are tedious and boring. And who in their right mind would bother investing their limited time and energy into doing something they may not particularly enjoy, especially when the promised rewards are so completely exaggerated?

Well, what if I told you that I had harnessed a groundbreaking physiological discovery to create a brief, innovative workout that renders old-fashioned cardiovascular exercise obsolete? And what if I boasted that my 20–25 minute routine will not only enable you to build the physique of your dreams, but that it will also induce hormonal modifications that slow down *aging*? If you learned anything from Dr. Dents and his bullfrog, you would probably demand that I back up my lofty claims with some (good) science. It's time to revisit our old friend evolution.

BACK TO THE GREAT REALITY CHECK

Although the first anatomically modern humans appeared just 50,000 years ago, our ancestors came down from the trees and stood up over 5 *million* years ago. Once our primate ancestors descended from the trees and became bipedal, they also grew larger, requiring more food for survival. However, because terrestrial living coincided with a relative *decrease* in food availability, ground-dwelling primates would have had to range over increasingly larger areas to meet their nutritional and energy requirements. Through natural selection, the mechanics of an upright posture evolved to favor endurance over speed, making bipedalism a highly effective adaptation for wide-range foraging.

Anthropologists maintain that early humans spent at least three hours walking ten to twelve miles each day in order to procure adequate food for survival. And they were able to do so without starving because, after 5 million years of fine-tuning, the physiology of walking had evolved to be as energy efficient as possible.

In other words, our survival as a species came to rely on our genetic propensity for extraordinary endurance during low- to moderate-intensity activities like brisk walking or slow jogging. Hence, activities that fall within the so-called "fat-burning zone" favor overall *energy conservation*. But if your goal is to shed unwanted body fat, the last thing you want to do is *conserve* energy. That being the case, wouldn't it seem logical to *avoid* exercising within the precise low-intensity aerobic zone that 5 million years of natural selection designed for *energy conservation*?

OLD SCHOOL CARDIO: AN EXERCISE IN FUTILITY

Everyone knows a cardio queen. She would sooner eat worms than miss her daily appointment with the treadmill. The funny thing is, most cardio queens don't look all that spectacular. In fact, she might be better off eating the worms—at least they're loaded with protein!

The old-school approach to weight loss and physical fitness emphasized lengthy sessions of moderate-intensity cardiovascular exercise. We were told to climb onto a treadmill, find the pace that corresponded to our aerobic "fat-burning" target heart rate, and march to nowhere for as long as we could tolerate the mind-numbing monotony of a human hamster wheel. Well, it turns out that although moderate-intensity aerobic exercise burns some fat *during* the actual activity, this brand of cardio has minimal impact on muscle toning and does almost nothing for increasing your metabolic rate. Don't get me wrong: Even low-intensity cardio is better than nothing. Previously sedentary individuals get results from just about any increase in activity level—at least for a little while. In the long run, however, the progress you can expect from moderate-intensity cardiovascular exercise is extremely limited. Plus it's about as exciting as watching the dust collect on your Bowflex.

The concept of an aerobic "fat burning zone" gained popularity in the early nineties, about the same time the anti-food group diet strategies were making everyone fat. The theoretical basis for the magical fat-burning zone derives from the premise that exercising at 60 to 70 percent of your maximal heart rate results in more total *lipid oxidation* (fat burning) than exercising at any other level of intensity. For most, this range, which is often referred to as the "target zone," corresponds to what would be a brisk walk or a slow jog. Like many theories, the notion of an ideal fat burning zone might look great on paper, but in practice, this brand of cardio is actually inefficient for promoting appreciable fat loss.

Why doesn't it work like it's supposed to?

Well, for starters, when you begin to exercise at an intensity corresponding to 65 percent of your maximum heart rate, only 30 to 40 percent of the total calories you burn derive from fat; the remainder come from muscle glycogen and blood glucose. As you continue to exercise at this intensity, you gradually consume muscle glycogen stores and fat starts to pick up the slack. After 30 minutes, fat oxidation represents about 50 percent of your total energy expenditure. After 90 minutes to two hours of sustained activity in your target zone, glycogen reservoirs become exhausted, and roughly two-thirds of calories burned are the direct result of fat oxidation.

In other words, if you were to burn 200 calories during a half-hour session of target zone aerobic exercise, less than 100 of those calories would actually come from fat. At that rate, it would take you over a month to lose just one pound of fat! Fortunately, the total number of calories burned as a result of exercising is a much better predictor of weight loss than the total fat oxidation that occurs during the activity.

Well, that's good news, especially if you decide to exceed your fat-burning target zone. Although a greater proportion of energy comes from fat oxidation when you exercise at low to moderate intensities, the total number of calories that you burn over time is greater when you exercise at higher intensities. Moreover, exercising at low to moderate intensities fails to evoke the physiological mechanisms that are most efficient for dispatching flab.

Fat-burning aside, the health benefits of low intensity cardio are minimal. For years, the same experts who devised those detestable food pyramids, aka the American Heart Association, advised everyone to walk for thirty minutes a day for good heart health. This, they insisted, was adequate to prevent heart disease and premature death. Well, apparently the American Heart Association based their exercise recommendations on the same nonexistent data they used to build their upside-down food pyramids. A recently published study that followed over 2,000 men for a decade has found that walking for 30 minutes a day does little if anything to maintain heart health and is totally ineffective for preventing cardiac death.

When it comes to improved body composition and heart health, the effectiveness of your exercise program relies on three separate factors:

1. The total calories you expend during your workout;

2. The muscle development that results from your workout;

3. The caloric *afterburn* you induce as a result of your workout.

If you want to build a firm, flab-free physique, the calories you expend during your workout may be the least significant of these three factors. For most, this is a very difficult concept to embrace because it flies in the face of everything you think you know about weight loss. In fact, most so-called weight loss experts still prescribe moderate intensity cardio within the fat-burning target zone as the most effective way to speed fat loss—despite cutting-edge research that contradicts this notion. Today, exercise physiologists are discovering that the most efficient way to induce progressive (and permanent!) fat loss isn't necessarily spending tedious hours in the fat-burning zone, but rather elevating metabolic rate around the clock—an endeavor best accomplished through activities that maximize both muscle toning and *excess post-exercise oxygen consumption (EPOC)*, otherwise known as caloric *afterburn*.

You see, exercise does not just burn calories *during* the activity; it also causes an increase in energy expenditure for up to two days *after* your workout. This increase in energy expenditure is reflected by elevated oxygen uptake: For every additional liter of oxygen consumed, approximately five extra calories are burned. Unlike low- to moderate-intensity aerobic exercise, which is fueled by a combination of fat and glucose, EPOC is fueled *exclusively* by fat oxidation. By comparing baseline (pre-exercise) oxygen consumption with post-exercise oxygen consumption, exercise physiologists can assess the extent of the EPOC generated by different forms of physical activity.

Researchers have been exploring this phenomenon for more than two decades. However, it is only recently that they have begun to appreciate the tremendous impact that manipulating different exercise variables can have on the magnitude and duration of caloric afterburn. Unfortunately, the majority of fitness trainers have never even heard of EPOC, and there are even fewer doctors and weight loss experts who understand the implications of exploiting it as a tool for improving body composition.

THE LEAN ESSENTIALS:

- Although a greater proportion of energy comes from fat oxidation when you exercise within the so-called fat-burning zone, the total number of calories that you burn over time is greater when you exercise at higher intensities.

- The overall number of calories you burn as a result of exercising is a much better predictor of weight loss than immediate fat oxidation (fat burning).

- For building a firm, flab-free physique, muscle toning and caloric afterburn are far more efficient than exercising within the "fat-burning zone."

ENTERING THE EPOC ZONE

Moderate intensity physical activities do not result in appreciable afterburn unless they are performed for extended periods of time. This is the primary reason that, until now, nobody has seriously considered exploiting EPOC for weight management. In order to elicit significant afterburn from target zone aerobic exercise, you would essentially have to run a marathon. Even if your schedule permitted running several marathons every week, the physical toll of doing so would destabilize your homeostasis and rapidly destroy your health. (Too much exercise is just as bad for you as too little!) Luckily, there are far more efficient and less tedious ways to induce substantial EPOC than lengthy sessions of cardio.

When researchers compared different forms of exercise to ascertain which was the best for maximizing EPOC, they quickly discovered that resistance training (weight lifting) and interval training (sprint-type activities) were enormously more effective for elevating post-exercise afterburn than moderate-intensity aerobic exercise. Both resistance and interval training have something in common: Unlike target zone cardio, which relies on a process known as *aerobic glycolysis,* weight lifting and sprints utilize *anaerobic glycolysis* for energy production.

Aerobic glycolysis burns both fat and glucose, and requires large amounts of oxygen. However, even if you are extremely fit, activities that elevate your heart rate above the magical fat-burning zone will eventually overcome your cardiovascular capabilities. For more intense, shorter duration activities like sprints, oxygen demands rapidly exceed oxygen supplies and an alternative method of energy production known as *anaerobic glycolysis* comes into play. Unlike aerobic glycolysis, anaerobic glycolysis does not require oxygen, nor does it burn much fat *during* the actual activity. However, anaerobic exercise produces substantial EPOC.

Ongoing research continues to explore the physiological mechanisms underlying the phenomenon of caloric afterburn. Most of the processes involved with short-term EPOC (up to one hour post-exercise) relate to the replenishment of oxygen and fuel stores, the removal of metabolic waste products, and transient elevations in ventilation (breathing), circulation (blood flow), and body temperature. However, very little is actually known about the specific physiological mechanisms responsible for the extended afterburn that can accelerate metabolic rate by 4 to 7 percent for up to two days following intense, anaerobic training. As investigators continue to unravel the complex hormonal relationships governing long-term EPOC, I predict that *growth hormone* will rise to the top of the list as one of the key players.

GROWTH HORMONE: YOUR UNTAPPED FOUNTAIN OF YOUTH AND FAT BURNING

In almost every area of homeostasis, when it comes to muscle toning and fat burning, women are at a distinct disadvantage compared to men. Testosterone, the primary male sex hormone, drives muscle development and helps men stay lean. On the other hand, estrogen, the primary female sex hormone, tends to increase the fat deposits on our buns, hips, and thighs. Women, however, have a secret weapon for fighting the battle of the bulge: *growth hormone.*

Growth hormone, also known as *somatotropin*, is synthesized and secreted by the pituitary gland, located at the base of the skull. Growth hormone is a major player in numerous metabolic processes. By stimulating the release of *insulin-like growth factor* (*IGF-1*) from the liver, growth hormone is indirectly responsible for long bone growth in children. In adults, the combined effects of growth hormone and IGF-1 do everything from reducing body fat, to promoting muscle tissue development, to preventing cosmetic symptoms of aging such as thinning skin.

The last two decades have witnessed considerable interest in administering *exogenous* (supplemental) growth hormone as a so-called therapy for aging. Unfortunately, scientific investigation has revealed that supplemental growth hormone often does more harm than good. In fact, there is evidence that growth hormone therapy actually *accelerates* certain aspects of aging and can reduce total life span. In contrast, raising one's *endogenous* (naturally occurring) levels of growth hormone through regular physical exertion remains one of our most potent weapons against the ravages of time as well as the threat of a flabby physique.

One of the most common casualties of aging is a healthy activity level, especially good old-fashioned get-your-heart-pounding-til-you're-out-of-breath exercise. Unfortunately, it's just this type of intense physical activity that is most effective for promoting growth hormone secretion. Cutting-edge research suggests that by adopting the type of high-intensity workout routine known to maximize natural growth hormone production, you can reduce the impact of many of the degenerative processes commonly associated with aging. For example, training strategies that increase circulating growth hormone also help prevent age-related reductions in bone density, skin thickness, and lean tissue (muscle) mass. In addition, these workouts promote the release of stored fat while blocking new fat storage. All of which is great news for your flab-free physique!

Increasing exercise intensity amplifies levels of circulating growth hormone regardless of gender. However, studies indicate that women have a significantly greater potential for harnessing exercise-induced increases in growth hormone production. Gender comparisons reveal that women not only secrete greater quantities of growth hormone in response to intense exercise, but that they do so more frequently than age-matched men. However, as with EPOC, certain types of exercise are much more efficient for amplifying our natural production of growth hormone. As fate would have it, the same anaerobic exercises that supercharge caloric afterburn are also best for increasing levels of circulating growth hormone.

Although intense weight lifting enhances both EPOC and growth hormone secretion, you do not have to lift heavy weights to optimize your workout results. Several studies have shown that circuit training, which utilizes relatively light resistances, can be just as effective at driving both EPOC and growth hormone release. Intuitively, circuit training might seem less intense than power training. However, circuit training calls for an increased number of repetitions per set. In addition, the rest periods between consecutive sets are short, typically on the order of thirty seconds or less. This may explain why the physiological responses to circuit training mimic high intensity, maximal effort interval training like all-out sprints.

THE LEAN ESSENTIALS:

- Increased levels of circulating growth hormone lead to reductions in body fat, increases in muscle tone and bone density, and may even prevent the cosmetic symptoms of aging.

- Women secrete greater quantities of growth hormone in response to intense exercise and they do so more frequently than age-matched men.

- Research indicates that intense circuit training is a great way to both harness EPOC and increase growth hormone secretion.

EXERCISING FOR A BEAUTIFUL BODY: MAXIMUM RESULTS IN MINIMUM TIME

The most efficient and effective exercise routine for building a fabulously firm physique harnesses your body's natural propensity for simultaneous fat burning and lean tissue development. This type of exercise program is a far cry from old school, fat-burning target-zone cardio.

As exercise physiologists are now discovering, the most efficient way to induce progressive (and permanent!) weight loss is to elevate metabolic rate around the clock—an endeavor best accomplished through a combination of resistance training and intense, short-duration exercise. Resistance training builds muscle and, as you learned in Chapter 1, a little muscle goes a long way toward increasing metabolic rate, caloric expenditure, and fat burning. Likewise, brief intervals of intense exercise induce a hormonal response that raises resting metabolic rate and increases overall fat burning for up to two days.

The whole trick to a fantastic, youthful physique resides in a routine that builds muscle while repeatedly elevating your heart rate out of the fat-burning target zone and into the out-of-breath anaerobic zone. For the fastest, most dramatic results possible, you want a workout that combines high energy expenditure *during* the training session with an even greater post-exercise afterburn to maximize caloric deficit. You also want a workout that stimulates muscle toning, optimizes EPOC, and increases growth hormone secretion.

On the other hand, most of us don't have several hours to devote to working out every day. Is it possible to bring all these variables together in a brief, manageable, exercise protocol?

It's not only possible; it's been done!

The *Ten Years Thinner* exercise program integrates the most powerful fat-burning, muscle-toning techniques for a total body workout that is as simple and efficient as physiologically possible. In essence, the workout routines utilize a fast-paced circuit of light weight lifting that burns calories, builds muscle, and elevates heart rate above the fat-burning target zone and into the out-of-breath anaerobic zone at regular intervals.

All the Benefits—Without the Risks

The most widely recognized methods for accessing the anaerobic zone currently involve intense, all-out efforts like sprinting. However, sprinting is a high-impact activity that can easily result in injury. The *Ten Years Thinner* exercise routines were carefully designed to be non-impact with minimal injury risk. Although these workouts mimic the anaerobic effects of interval training, injury risk is no greater than it would be for a basic circuit training program. The specific movements that are intended to drive your heart rate into the breathless anaerobic zone were chosen expressly for their simplicity. Even if you are a phys ed flunky who hasn't broken a sweat since high school gym class, after one or two *Ten Years Thinner* training sessions you will not find any of the movements difficult to execute.

Don't worry if it's been a long time since you got yourself out of breath! You will only be required to exercise at a high intensity for very brief intervals throughout the 20- to 25-minute routines. Because these workouts were designed to exploit progressive conditioning, even someone who is currently sedentary and out of shape will be able to do them successfully. To put it simply, the exertion required to elevate your heart rate into the anaerobic zone is directly proportional to your level of fitness. So, the more out of shape you are, the less you will need to exert yourself. As your conditioning improves, you will progress gradually, at your own pace. However, your perceived level of exertion never has to increase.

Regardless of your current fitness level, the *Ten Years Thinner* exercise program will provide rapid, tangible results that are guaranteed to keep you motivated on your journey to a firm, youthful physique.

THE LEAN ESSENTIALS:

- You will burn more calories during a twenty-minute *Ten Years Thinner* exercise routine than you would if you had instead spent thirty minutes speed walking in the fat-burning zone.

- The *Ten Years Thinner* workouts use circuits of light resistance training to tone all your muscles, maximize caloric afterburn, and enhance growth hormone secretion.

- The *Ten Years Thinner* exercise routines will flatten your stomach, lift your butt, thin your thighs, tone your torso, and supercharge your metabolism for continuous, around-the-clock fat incineration.

———— ✦✦✦✦✦ ————

"The *Ten Years Thinner* meal plan was more than satisfying.
I never felt hungry or deprived, and within two weeks,
I saw noticeable changes in my body." — KIM, 39

"The *Ten Years Thinner* meal plan isn't a diet.
It's just a different way of eating,
a healthy way that works!" — DARLENE, 43

"In terms of both time and effort, the *Ten Years Thinner*
dietary guidelines actually made it easier for
me to cook for myself and my family. Rather than
trying to avoid unhealthy ingredients, I was able to
focus on healthy ones." — JILLIAN, 38

"In two weeks I dropped two belt sizes and
gained lean muscle." — CHRISTOPHER, 34

"I am never hungry on the diet, and I have extra
energy to keep up with my two-year-old." — MELISSA, 36

"This program has totally changed how I think about food.
The great part is how easy it is to follow.
By the end of six weeks, it's second nature." — CATHY, 31

"Being a typical guy who's never really dieted, but who's
sat on the sidelines as diets have come and gone, I think to
call this program a 'diet' is a misnomer. A diet is something you
start and stop. This program isn't about dieting; this program
is about learning how to eat properly." — MATT, 38

———— ✦✦✦✦✦ ————

CHAPTER 8

The Ten Years Thinner Diet

Way back in the Introduction, I made a solemn promise to you that the *Ten Years Thinner* program would not entail deprivation, suffering, cravings, or mathematical calculations. And I meant it! It will not take you long to get the hang of eating for stable homeostasis and a revved metabolism. If you read the last seven chapters in their intended order, you will have no trouble understanding the basic principles that govern the diet, and you will have an easy time following it.

Take a moment now to familiarize yourself with the contents of Appendices A to D. Appendices A and B summarize the *Ten Years Thinner* program on a week-by-week basis and include extensive food and beverage lists. Appendix C contains compliance forms and a progress sheet for self-monitoring. Although completing these forms is optional, I highly recommend filling them out as you proceed through the six-week program. Most of my test subjects agreed that the compliance forms helped keep them on track, and everyone found it motivating to record the changes in their physiques as the inches melted away.

To help make the transition to healthy eating as effortless as possible, Appendix D contains a collection of quick, easy recipes for every week of the program. As you will soon realize, cooking meals according to the *Ten Years Thinner* guidelines is no more arduous or time consuming than just plain cooking meals. In fact, the one thing that all my test subjects emphasized during their exit interviews was how easy it was to prepare meals without spending any extra time in the kitchen. Many of them also expressed relief at not having to make two different meals, one for themselves and one for their families.

All the recipes in this book, many of which were donated by former test subjects, were chosen specifically for their simplicity and short preparation times. Hopefully, they will provide you with inspiration for your own culinary experiments. Even if you ignore the recipes completely, you can still be one hundred percent compliant with the *Ten Years Thinner* program simply by adhering to the dietary guidelines outlined below and choosing all the foods for your meals from the appropriate food and beverage lists.

THE RATIONALE BEHIND THE DIET

The *Ten Years Thinner* program is organized into two different phases, each of three weeks' duration. Part of the rationale behind this biphasic system is that it permits you the opportunity to identify food sensitivities of which you might not be aware. As you know, many of the foods in our modern, Western diet are not necessarily good for us. Specifically, dairy products and grains did not play a significant role in our diet until very recently in our evolutionary history. As a result, many people are physiologically ill equipped to digest and absorb these foods in a way that keeps systemic inflammation in check and promotes stable homeostasis. Because efficient fat burning and extended longevity rely so heavily on stable homeostasis, identifying food sensitivities is a vital first step toward both sustainable weight loss and maintaining a youthful appearance.

If every food sensitivity resulted in hives or anaphylaxis, it would be a simple matter to identify and eliminate those foods from your diet. However, food sensitivities can evoke such a wide spectrum of unpredictable symptoms, it is often very difficult to draw a connection between the food and the reaction it causes. Many (if not most!) people eat foods that are slowly destroying their health. Roughly half of the test subjects who participated in my *Ten Years Thinner* clinical trials discovered they were at least moderately sensitive to various foods. The most common adverse reactions (low energy, fatigue, and mild joint stiffness) occurred most often when these individuals resumed grain consumption.

Just a Few Examples

After developing painful arthritis in his knees, Luke, an elite-level cyclist, was forced to stop racing. His arthritis worsened over time. Then, after a six-year hiatus from virtually all strenuous activity, Luke stopped eating wheat for a month and the pain disappeared! Since eliminating wheat from his diet, Luke, now 39, is once again racing mountain bikes at a highly competitive level. *And his thinning hair is growing back!*

Carry, a 36-year-old woman who'd struggled with acne since puberty, realized that she consistently broke out every time she ate cheese. She now eschews cow cheese, substituting goat or soy-based cheeses, and her skin is completely clear.

One of my biggest weight loss success stories, a 34-year-old woman named Lisa who had a formidable family history of obesity, diabetes, and heart disease (her sister underwent quadruple bypass at the shockingly young age of 42), discovered she was so sensitive to high glycemic index foods that even adding a few semi-sweet chocolate chips to her snack mix, or having a single slice of bread with her meal, caused mood swings, sugar cravings, and made her energy levels plummet for up to two days.

Another woman, Christine, a 43-year-old mother of two, found that eliminating milk from her diet cured the debilitating menstrual cramps she'd suffered since adolescence. *And the list goes on and on!*

One of the best ways to assess potential food sensitivities is to completely eliminate dubious items from your diet for a brief test period. After this cleansing phase, it's easier to recognize adverse reactions to questionable foods when they are reintroduced to your diet.

The *Ten Years Thinner* dietary elimination/reintroduction schedule proceeds as follows:

1. For the first two weeks of the *Ten Years Thinner* program,
    all legumes, soy-based foods, dairy, grains, and other high glycemic
    index carbs (potatoes, dried fruit, fruit juice, alcohol, etc.) are off limits.

2. At the beginning of week three, legumes are reintroduced.

3. At the beginning of week four, dairy and soy-based foods are reintroduced.

4. At the beginning of week five, select grains and other high glycemic index carbs are reintroduced.

5. After week six, you may resume drinking alcohol.

Beyond identifying food sensitivities, the temporary elimination of all grains and other high glycemic index (HGI) carbs from your diet serves another important purpose. The overwhelming majority of North Americans are at least mildly addicted (physically as well as psychologically) to HGI carbohydrates. It's your sugar addiction that is responsible for most of your unhealthy food cravings. Eschewing HGI carbs for a period of four weeks will break your sugar addiction and enable you to kick your HGI carb habit once and for all. Do not be alarmed if you experience mild headaches or are unusually fatigued for the first day or two; these are typical withdrawal symptoms for someone suffering an HGI carb addiction. Rest assured, your energy levels should return to normal by the end of the first week, and will likely be higher than ever before by the end of the second. When these foods are reintroduced in limited quantities at the beginning of week 5, you will no longer be tempted to overindulge.

GENERAL GUIDELINES

There are five fundamental guidelines you will be asked to follow for the duration of the *Ten Years Thinner* program. By the end of the six weeks, each one of these simple rules of healthy eating will be a natural, effortless part of your day-to-day existence.

#1: Eat Frequently

The *Ten Years Thinner* meal plan calls for the daily consumption of three mandatory meals, two mandatory between-meal snacks, and an optional pre-bedtime snack.

You might be worried about how your body will react to so much food. Don't be! Eating frequently does *not* make you fat. On the contrary, the more frequently you eat, the faster you'll build a firm, flab-free physique. There are several reasons for this.

First, the heat generated by your body during the ingestion, digestion, and absorption of food causes a temporary increase in your metabolic rate. This phenomenon, known as the *thermic effect* of a meal, is most pronounced during the initial 90 minutes after you eat. The more frequently you have a small meal or snack, the more thermic effect your body generates, and the more calories you burn as a direct result of eating. In other words, someone who typically eats five 300-calorie meals per day will have a racier metabolism (and will burn more fat between meals) than someone who eats three 500-calorie meals instead. Second, the hungrier you are when you finally break your fast and have a meal, the greater the likelihood that you will overeat. And finally, the longer you make your body wait between meals, the less efficient it becomes at burning fat, and the more muscle tissue you sacrifice to glucose production. As you know, when it comes to building a firm, youthful physique, muscle breakdown is the kiss of death.

What about the pre-bedtime snack? Haven't you always heard that eating around bedtime makes you fat? Well, it doesn't have to. In fact, by exploiting your body's natural hormonal rhythms, eating before sleeping can actually help you get leaner even faster.

As you know from Chapter 7, growth hormone speeds fat loss, blocks fat gain, enhances exercise recovery and muscle toning, and has anti-aging properties that include increased skin elasticity. Although anaerobic exercise raises growth hormone production, the majority of growth hormone release occurs at night while you sleep. Protein ingestion raises serum amino acid levels, which, in turn, stimulate additional growth hormone release. So, by consuming protein foods shortly before bedtime, you will maximize natural growth hormone secretion while you sleep. If you typically finish your last meal more than three hours before retiring, you should have an additional protein snack about an hour prior to hitting the hay. Your firm body will thank you in the morning!

#2: Drink Frequently

The *Ten Years Thinner* meal plan calls for the consumption of at least 60 ounces (about two liters) of fluid per day, or about 10 to 12 ounces with every meal and snack. This volume should be *in addition to* whatever fluids you drink when exercising.

Up to this point, I've talked a lot about macronutrients, but I've made no mention of the importance of adequate fluid intake. Don't let this fool you into thinking that proper hydration is any less important to a stable homeostasis and lean body composition than proper nutrition. It's every bit as important; it's just a whole lot simpler!

Water aids the liver and kidneys in the detoxification of poisons and the elimination of wastes from the body. Without sufficient fluid intake, dehydration impedes organ function, hinders homeostasis, and slows metabolism. You read right—dehydration contributes to a sluggish metabolism, which contributes to a flabby physique! Generous fluid intake, on the other hand, is associated with a lower risk of heart disease, younger-looking skin, and a leaner body composition. Plus, water is an excellent diuretic; the more you drink, the less water you retain.

Because we do not feel thirsty until we are already in a state of mild dehydration, it's best to drink enough to *avoid* rather than to quench thirst. This is especially true just prior to your work out when water losses will increase as a result of increased perspiration. Proper hydration during intense exercise translates to higher blood volume and enhanced oxygen exchange in the lungs. In other words, your cardiovascular system doesn't have to work as hard to get oxygen-rich blood to active muscle tissue and you enjoy a more comfortable and productive training session. Brief water breaks are both permitted and encouraged throughout the exercise routines.

#3: Include a Full Serving of
Lean Protein with Every Meal

As you know, adequate protein, consumed frequently throughout the day, is absolutely vital to muscle toning and fat burning. It might interest you to learn that protein has roughly three times the thermic effect of either fat or carbohydrate. That means the more protein your meal contains, the more calories you will burn digesting your food.

Referring back to Chapter 2, you might recall that a fabulously firm physique requires about three-quarters of a gram of lean protein per pound of ideal body weight per day. Each of your two or three daily snacks will include about 10 grams of protein. So, if your ideal weight falls between 120 and 160 pounds, you would need to consume roughly 20 to 30 grams (80–120 calories) of protein with each of your three meals.

Well, I promised you back in Chapter 1 that you would never have to use complicated calculations to comply with the *Ten Years Thinner* meal plan. There is an easy, foolproof method for estimating portion size without resorting to time-consuming and inconvenient practices like weighing your food at every single meal. In fact, all you need to do is look at your hand! The volume of cooked protein on your plate should approximate the volume of your hand—fingers included.

#4: Include at Least One Serving of Fruit and/or Vegetables with Every Meal

The health benefits of high consumption of fresh fruits and vegetables are legion. The *Ten Years Thinner* meal plan includes a minimum of one serving of fruit and/or vegetables with each of your three meals. To estimate what constitutes a serving, just go straight to the end of your wrist. Use your fist as a gauge: One serving of fruit equals approximately one fist; one serving of vegetables (or salad) equals approximately two fists.

Realize that these are *minimal* recommendations. Feel free to eat as much fruit and as many vegetables as your heart desires. Fruits and vegetables will never make you fat! In fact, I recommend starting every meal with a small salad. The fiber content of your salad fixings will begin to provide you with a feeling of satiety even before you start on your main course.

#5: Cook Exclusively with Cold-Pressed Extra-Virgin Olive Oil

As you know from Chapter 3, fat plays a vital role in signaling your brain that you're full so you are not tempted to overeat. In addition, fat slows the absorption of carbohydrates and functionally lowers the glycemic index of a meal. For these reasons alone, it is important to include moderate amounts of fat with every meal and snack.

Even the leanest protein foods generally contribute some fat to your meal. However, with the exception of whole eggs, it's just not enough. Fortunately, the nuts you will be snacking on between your meals, plus the extra-virgin olive oil you will be using to cook your meals, will provide ample amounts of the healthy fats your body needs in order to maintain a well-oiled homeostasis and a revved, fat-burning metabolism.

As you know, the polyunsaturated vegetable oils once thought to promote good heart health do anything but. This is partly due to their high pro-inflammatory omega-6 fatty acid content, and partly due to the multiple double bonds that occur within their carbon chains. Multiple double bonds make polyunsaturated vegetable oils far less stable than olive oil, which is comprised predominantly of monounsaturated fatty acids containing only one double bond. Unlike polyunsaturated vegetable oils, olive oil is unlikely to undergo the chemical reactions that produce cancer-promoting, artery-clogging free radicals.

In addition, cold-pressed extra-virgin olive oil boasts some truly astounding functional properties that make it far and away the best choice for promoting a balanced homeostasis and a revved, fat-burning, physique-firming metabolism. Research demonstrates that the consumption of olive oil fights inflammatory processes, effectively combating obesity, many forms of cancer, hypertension, and heart disease. Moreover, cold-pressed extra-virgin olive oil contains a rare and extremely powerful antioxidant phytochemical known as *hydroxytyrosol*. By preventing the oxidation of certain proteins intrinsic to hair, nail, and skin health, hydroxytyrosol makes hair softer and shinier, renders nails stronger and more resistant to breakage, and helps prevent the cosmetic symptoms of aging skin. Perhaps even more importantly, hydroxytyrosol protects fish oil supplements from oxidation by free radicals. For this reason, I recommend that you always take your omega-3 fish oil supplements with a meal that includes some olive oil.

THE LEAN ESSENTIALS

- For the duration of the *Ten Years Thinner* program, you must eat three meals and two snacks per day.

- You must drink 10 to 12 ounces of clear fluid with each of your meals and snacks.

- Each meal must include one serving of lean protein.

- Each meal must include *at least* one serving of fruit and/or vegetables.

- All cooking must be done using cold-pressed, extra virgin olive oil.

THE TEN YEARS THINNER DIET: PHASE 1 (WEEKS 1–3)

(For Food Lists, see Appendix A.)

A Word on Protein Foods

All the protein foods listed for Phase 1 (see Appendix A) are relatively lean, deriving 20 to 30 percent of their calories from fat. This fat content approximates the leanness of the wild game that humans evolved eating. The only exception to this rule is whole eggs.

Whole eggs (yolk plus white) derive about 40 percent of their total calories from fat, with virtually all of the fat existing within the egg yolk. However, contrary to what you might have been led to believe, eating egg yolks will not impact your cholesterol levels in a way that promotes vessel disease. Whole eggs are an excellent source of heart-healthy monounsaturated fat, high quality protein, vitamins, and minerals. But not all eggs are created equal! Free range eggs come from happier, healthier chickens and their yolks contain healthier ratios of fatty acids. If you opt *not* to use free range eggs, you should discard half of the yolks. For example, rather than a three-egg omelet, use four whites and two yolks.

At the beginning of week 3, your list of protein options expands to include fattier cuts of poultry and low-fat processed meats like cold cuts and sausage. To determine if your cold cuts or sausages qualify as low fat, simply check to make sure that the total fat content doesn't exceed about 35 percent of total calories. In other words, there should be at least 4 grams of protein for every gram of fat.

Fruits, Vegetables, and Legumes

Frozen fruits and vegetables may be substituted for fresh fare. Fruits and vegetables are frozen at the peak of ripeness when they are loaded with vitamins, minerals, antioxidant nutrients, and phytochemicals. As a result, frozen fruit and vegetables may contain even more nutrients than fresh fruits and vegetables that were harvested green and left to ripen during their long voyage to the produce section of your grocery store.

However, with the exception of legumes (peas, beans, and peanuts), dried, canned, and jarred fruits and vegetables should be avoided because these processes increase the glycemic index of the food item. (Limited amounts of dried fruit will be reintroduced during Phase 2.) Moreover, the processing and preserving techniques that make canning possible destroy nutrients and often involve the addition of unhealthy amounts of sodium.

Starting at the beginning of week 3, legumes (peas, beans, and peanuts) will be added to your food list along with fruits and vegetables (see Appendix A). Although legumes boast many health benefits, they were largely absent from the prehistoric diet, and some people will notice they are sensitive to these food items. If you elect to use canned legumes, I recommend first rinsing them with cold water to reduce their sodium content.

Snacking: Go Nuts for Nuts

You are probably going to enjoy snacking on the *Ten Years Thinner* program. Sure, there may have to be some changes. For now, there won't be any more cookies, chips, ice cream, or popcorn, but you do get to eat lots of nuts! For the next three weeks, your midmorning and midafternoon snack will consist of up to half a cup of shelled, mixed nuts (a couple generous handfuls) plus one serving of fresh fruit (see Appendix A). This snack is delicious, nutritious, filling, convenient, totally portable, and requires absolutely no preparation. (Unless, of course, you plan to do the shelling yourself.)

Nuts are high in protein, fiber, and healthy monounsaturated fats. They are also loaded with vitamins, minerals, and antioxidant phytochemicals. Nuts are guaranteed to prevent those pesky, between-meal cravings that have been known to send so many well-intentioned dieters sneaking off to the candy machine for a Ding Dong or a bag of chips.

While it's true that nuts *are* high in both fat and calories, snacking on nuts will not make *you* fat! On the contrary, studies indicate that people who eat nuts on a regular basis are far *less* likely to be overweight, hypertensive, or diabetic. In fact, people who eat a handful of nuts at least five times a week cut their risk for having a heart attack *in half*. Other research suggests that nuts improve cholesterol profiles, decrease cardiovascular risks, prevent cancer, keep your skin looking younger, and increase muscle retention for a leaner body composition. So, don't be afraid to go a little nuts for nuts.

About the Beverages

In addition to water, the beverage list for Phase 1 (see Appendix A) includes sparkling water, green tea, and herbal teas. I recommend using lemon, lime, or fresh berry juice to spice up plain or sparkling water and hot or iced tea.

Although up to three cups of coffee or black tea a day are also permitted, these beverages do not count toward the 60 ounces of clear fluid you should be drinking on a daily basis. Coffee and black tea both contain significant amounts of caffeine and theophylline. While these compounds can elevate metabolism and spark additional fat burning, they also function as diuretics and tend to increase water loss in the urine.

Iced green tea (three tea bags per two quarts of water) is a light, tasty alternative to plain water. Moreover, green tea is loaded with health-promoting antioxidants and anti-inflammatory polyphenols. Numerous investigations demonstrate an association between green tea consumption and lower LDL cholesterol, diminished LDL cholesterol oxidation, and decreased incidence of heart disease, heart attack, and stroke. Other studies indicate that green tea consumption decreases symptoms of arthritis; improves kidney, liver, and pancreatic function; prevents and fights many forms of cancer; and can even help protect your skin and eyes from sun damage. And great news for your firm physique: According to a rapidly growing body of research data, green tea represents a potent, natural fat burner.

Although it contains a moderate dose of caffeine, other compounds unique to green tea inhibit caffeine's harsh side effects. As a result, green tea is unlikely to make you feel edgy or nervous the way a strong cup of coffee can. However, green tea can make you feel invigorated. If you are prone to insomnia, taper your intake of green tea late in the day.

You will notice that the beverage list for Phase 1 does not include any fruit juice. This deliberate omission probably strikes you as peculiar, especially after I spent the better part of Chapter 4 extolling the many virtues of fruit. Let me explain: Fruit juice is basically fruit robbed of its fiber. Most juice that comes in a carton has also been processed and stripped of vital nutrients like vitamins, minerals, and antioxidants. And even though fructose (fruit sugar) has a much lower glycemic index than glucose, fruit juice is calorically dense and in the absence of fiber it causes a rapid rise in blood glucose. Limited amounts of fruit juice are permitted during weeks 4 to 6 as part of a healthy meal or as a smoothie ingredient. But if you're into juicing because of all its purported health benefits, it's time to find a new hobby.

A Word on Condiments

During Phase 1, you may season your food with as much salt, pepper and other spices, garlic, horseradish, vinegar, pickles, olive oil and vinegar or vinaigrette salad dressing, hot sauce, lemon juice, sesame seeds, salsa, and mustard as you want (see Appendix A). However, for the next three weeks, you must avoid all mayo, ketchup, BBQ sauce, tartar sauce, creamy salad dressing, soy sauce, tomato sauce, cocktail sauce, sugar, honey, and peanut butter.

THE TEN YEARS THINNER DIET:
PHASE 2 (WEEKS 4–6)

(For Food Lists, see Appendix B.)

Until now, with the exception of nuts, all the items on your food lists have had unlimited consumption recommendations. In other words, you were advised to eat *at least* one serving of protein, plus *at least* one serving of fresh fruit and/or vegetables at each of your three meals. And, if you felt like it, you were welcome to eat more. This will never change. Now, however, as foods are reintroduced, some will have recommended upper limits for consumption. These restricted items include most dairy foods, soy foods, and HGI carbs like bread, cereal, potatoes, fruit juice, dried fruit, and chocolate. All restricted foods and their upper limits are clearly indicated in Appendix B.

New Protein Foods

At the beginning of week 4, your list of protein options expands to include egg and whey protein supplements. For decades, egg protein was considered the gold standard of protein supplementation. And to its credit, egg protein boasts a solid, overall amino acid profile and is extremely well absorbed and utilized by exercising muscles. Unfortunately, egg protein has been known to spawn the foulest-smelling farts ever produced by land-dwelling life forms. For this reason, I usually recommend trying whey protein products instead.

High quality whey protein is essentially lactose free, contains near zero HGI carbs, and boasts an extremely high concentration of essential amino acids. In addition, whey protein has been experimentally shown to boost immune function. According to research, whey supplementation helps combat bacterial infections and increases the immune response caused by exposure to carcinogens. In several studies, whey was found to inhibit the growth of tumor cells. Whey protein has also been experimentally shown to stimulate the anabolic hormone IGF-1, which is known to help prevent bone loss and osteoporosis.

The Reintroduction of Dairy and Soy

At the beginning of week 4, in addition to the mandatory serving of animal protein, you may now also have up to 100 calories worth of dairy or soy-based foods with each of your three meals (see Appendix B). However, unless these new food items actually appear on the protein list (as several dairy foods do), they cannot be substituted for a serving of lean protein. For hard cheeses, 100 calories generally corresponds to approximately two fingers worth. Whenever possible, choose fat-free, low-fat, or reduced fat versions.

Grains and Other HGI Carbs

At the beginning of week 5, select grains and HGI carbs are reintroduced. None of these food options (including corn, potatoes, or dried fruit) should be substituted for the mandatory servings of fresh fruit and/or vegetables. Moreover, all of these new food items are to be consumed in *limited* quantities as described on the food lists in Appendix B.

Restricted Condiments:
The Two-Tablespoon Rule

Phase 2 will see the introduction of many new condiments. In addition to the growing list of unrestricted condiments, you will find a number of restricted items like creamy dressings and honey. For most restricted condiments, you should follow the two-tablespoon rule, limiting their use to two tablespoons per meal (see Appendix B).

Advanced Snack Mix

Starting at the beginning of week 4, in addition to or instead of snack mix and fruit, you may have a single serving of plain yogurt at snack times. Starting at the beginning of week 5, you may include up to two ounces of dried fruit or chocolate chips with your snack mix.

Fruit Juice

Starting at the beginning of week 4, you may have up to 1 cup (8 ounces) of fruit juice per day. Starting at the beginning of week 5, you may have up to 2 cups (16 ounces) of fruit juice per day. To functionally lower the glycemic index of fruit juice, you should only drink it with meals and/or as part of a protein smoothie recipe.

LISTEN TO YOUR BODY!

During Phase 2, you will be required to pay very careful attention to your physiology. If you notice that your energy levels plummet every time you eat potatoes, or that your joints ache the day after you eat wheat-based foods, or that you tend to break out when you eat chocolate, don't ignore these obvious signs of disturbed homeostasis. Accept that you probably shouldn't be eating these foods and take the necessary steps to eliminate them from your diet on a more permanent basis.

THE LEAN ESSENTIALS

(For full food lists, refer to Appendices A and B.)

- For the first two weeks of the *Ten Years Thinner* program, all legumes, soy-based foods, dairy, grains, and other high glycemic carbs are off limits.

- At the beginning of week 3, legumes are reintroduced.

- At the beginning of week 4, dairy and soy-based foods are reintroduced.

- At the beginning of week 5, select grains and other HGI carbs are reintroduced.

- After week 6, you may resume drinking alcohol.

- *Listen to your body!* If the reintroduction of any food corresponds to an adverse reaction, this is a red flag for disturbed homeostasis.

———— ✦✦✦✦✦ ————

"The exercise program doesn't leave you exhausted for
the rest of the day or make you sore for the next day.
Even with all the things I have on my plate,
this program was easy for me to follow. So I ask my friends,
what's stopping you?" — JILLIAN, 38

"My arms and legs were stronger and noticeably
more toned with every passing week." — LAURIE, 43

"I love that I can do the workouts at home. I work full time and
I have two kids, a two-year-old and a five-year-old, so time
is at a premium for me. My kids like to do the exercises with me,
only without the weights. It makes things fun, and it teaches
them that exercise is an important part of life." — DARLENE, 43

"I would definitely recommend this program to my friends.
I think if they were to try it for three weeks and
see the results, they'd be hooked." — COLLEEN, 43

"I really like that the exercise routine works your
entire body in under half an hour." — FRANCOISE, 26

———— ✦✦✦✦✦ ————

CHAPTER 9

The Ten Years Thinner Workout

T ake a moment and have a good, long look at yourself in your bathroom mirror. The transformation that your body is about to undergo will be more dramatic than you might imagine. In as little as two or three days from now, you will begin to feel changes in your physique. In as little as a week, you will begin to see a difference in the bathroom mirror. Many of my fitness clients have found it fun and motivating to take progressive before and after pictures, or measure their waist, hips, and chest every week or ten days as they advance through the initial six weeks of their diet and exercise program. (Appendix C contains a form you can fill out to track your progress.) If you plan to take a couple of snapshots, or record your shrinking girth, don't wait until tomorrow to document your starting point; do it now, *before* your first workout.

And whatever you do, *don't* become a slave to your bathroom scale! Your scale will not give you an accurate picture of your changing body composition. Using your weight as a way to gauge your progress toward a firm physique is like referring to last week's weather report to determine if it will rain over the coming weekend. (It's the sort of thing Dr. Dents might do.)

First of all, day-to-day alterations in body weight are an imprecise method for assessing fat loss. About the only thing you might learn by jumping on the scale every morning is how much water you happen to be retaining relative to the day

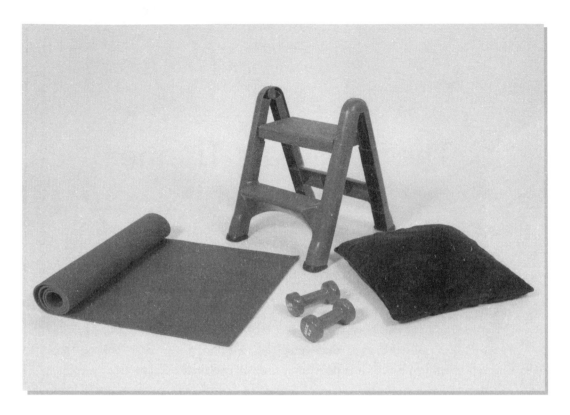

The equipment.

before. The volume of fluid your body holds is influenced by countless variables from salt intake to simply being female. Increases in water retention commonly cause daily weight fluctuations of three to five pounds, which is more fat mass than you could possibly gain or lose in a 24-hour period.

Furthermore, it's important to remind yourself that one of your main objectives is to actually *gain* some muscle tissue. Much of the success of this program resides in the fact that lean tissue is extremely metabolically active, and the additional muscle you're building will ultimately increase around-the-clock fat burning. However, because lean tissue is so much denser than fatty tissue, overall weight loss is an inaccurate gauge of true progress.

When you adopt the eating and exercising habits described in *Ten Years Thinner*, it's not unusual to drop an impressive amount of weight very rapidly during the first week or two, only to find yourself hovering at the same body weight for the next week or two. Be aware that this weight plateau has nothing in common with the dreaded weight plateau I mentioned in Chapter 1. The vast majority of fad diet disciples are disappointed to see their weight stabilize long before they have achieved their fat loss goals. This is because most fad diets still employ defective weight loss strategies like severe caloric or carbohydrate restriction, which, as you know, lead to muscle loss, metabolic slowing, and eventually, more fat gain.

If you experience a temporary weight plateau while following the *Ten Years Thinner* program, it simply means you have entered a passing phase where you are building lean tissue at roughly the same rate (ounce for ounce) that you are shedding fat. Don't be discouraged by a temporary weight plateau. As long as you stick to the program, you will continue to lose unwanted body fat and inches even if your overall weight may remain relatively unchanged for a week or two. Whether you're losing pounds and inches, or just plain inches, the *Ten Years Thinner* program will melt the fat away to reveal a whole new, shapely you.

So, please take my advice and scale down on the weigh-ins. In fact, if I were you, I would take that evil instrument of psychological torture (otherwise known as your bathroom scale) straight out to the garage and leave it to do what it does best: sit on top of your Bowflex while they both collect dust.

THE LEAN ESSENTIALS:

- DON'T become a slave to your bathroom scale! Changes in body weight do not accurately reflect changes in body composition.

- DON'T become discouraged if you hit a weight plateau. As long as you stick to the meal plan and exercise program, you will continue to lose body fat and inches even if your overall weight remains temporarily unchanged.

GENERAL GUIDELINES

By applying the basic concepts that were introduced in Chapter 7, the *Ten Years Thinner* exercise routines will ease you into your workout program. Twenty minutes a day is all it will take to get you hooked! Firming and toning aside, two to three weeks from now, you will notice improved strength and coordination, increased energy and self-confidence, and an elevated mood. And the best part? These simple but effective exercises can be performed by virtually anyone—even if you haven't broken a sweat since high school gym class. And you won't need to join a fitness club, spend a fortune on exercise equipment, or relegate yourself to tedious hours on a human hamster wheel to see and feel results in about a week.

The Phase 1 workout consists of twelve sets of exercises, done back to back, with little or no rest between. The twelve exercises comprising the Phase 1 workout are roughly divided into three groups of similar exercises. Each group consists of an "exercise quartet," four different movements, which include:

1. a lower body or combined lower and upper body exercise

2. an upper body exercise

3. another lower body or combined exercise

4. an abdominal exercise

This pattern is intended to periodically spike your heart rate while providing a balanced, full-body workout that will only take about 20 minutes to complete. Although none of the movements are high impact or complicated, you *will* be pushing yourself into the out-of-breath anaerobic zone a total of four times during the 20-minute period. If you are sedentary, obese, and/or suffer from any serious medical condition for which you are currently under a doctor's care, including type 2 diabetes, hypertension, or any known heart disease, you should consult your physician before attempting these exercise routines.

THE TEN YEARS THINNER WORKOUT

Step 1: Preparing Your Workout Area

To make exercising as fun and convenient as possible, it's helpful to do a quick walk-through before you tackle your first workout. Remember, you will be taking little to no time between sets, so it is best to familiarize yourself with all the exercises and plan your route ahead of time.

DO post the appropriate exercise routine on a wall (see Appendices A and B) where you can refer to it quickly and easily. Don't trust your memory! The order of the specific movements is very important, and memory retrieval can be unreliable when you are engaged in strenuous activities.

DO have water available to you at all times. You are encouraged to drink a full glass about an hour before you begin and a couple of sips between movements if you become thirsty.

DO listen to music. Studies have shown that music can decrease perceived exertion and propel you through a physically demanding routine. In fact, listening to motivating beats may increase your ability to perform anaerobically. So by all means, crank your favorite tunes.

DO NOT watch television during your workout. If you have the spare energy to pay attention to a sit-com, you aren't pushing yourself hard enough.

Step 2: The Warm Up

A "cold" muscle feels stiff and weak and, relative to a warm muscle, it *is* stiff and weak. Similarly, tendons and ligaments will accommodate more stretch prior to injury when they are warmed up. Before you begin your workout, take three to five minutes and engage in alternating-leg knee-ups and arm windmills to increase the blood flow to your extremities and raise your core and peripheral body temperature.

Step 3: The Exercise Routine

The Phase 1 workouts consist of 12 sets of exercises to be completed in the order listed below:

	Recommended Number of Repetitions	
	Week 1	*Weeks 2 and 3*
1. Step-ups	10–15/leg	15–20/leg
2. Push-ups	10–20	20–30
3. Lunge-curls	10–15/leg	15–20/leg
4. Squeeze-crunches	15–20	20–30
5. Squat-presses	15–20	20–30
6. Rows	15–20	20–30
7. Squat-raises	15–20	20–30
8. Squeeze-side-crunches	7–10/side	10–15/side
9. Sissy-squats	15–20	20–30
10. Bench-dips	10–20	20–30
11. Calf-raises	15–20	20–30
12. Squeeze-crunches	15–20	20–30

Workout Schedule for Week 1 (Days 1–7)

Day 1 and 2	Week 1 Routine
Day 3	Rest
Days 4, 5, and 6	Week 1 Routine
Day 7	Rest
Day 8	Begin Week 2 and 3 Routine

The compliance form for Week 1 (see Appendix C) lists the appropriate exercise routine with rest days included.

Workout Schedule for Weeks 2 and 3 (Days 8–21)

Four days of training, followed by one day off

The compliance forms for Weeks 2 and 3 (see Appendix C) list the appropriate exercise routine with rest days included.

On pages 120–149, you will find an illustrated explanation of each exercise. The week 1 routine utilizes exactly the same exercises as the weeks 2 and 3 routine. The only differences between the two routines are the number of recommended repetitions per set, and the number of recommended days off between your training sessions.

The number of recommended repetitions per set is a basic guideline. If you cannot do the minimum number, this is OK. You will gain strength and stamina over the coming weeks as your conditioning improves. On the other hand, if you can easily do more than the maximum number of recommended repetitions, then it's time to raise the height of the step, move on to a more advanced version of the exercise (there are novice and regular versions of push-ups, bench-dips, and sissy-squats), or increase the denomination of your soup cans/dumbbells by a pound or two. For different exercises, you may find you need different size dumbbells. For example, most people find they prefer a slightly heavier weight for squat-presses than for squat-raises.

Step 4: Post-Workout Stretching Routine

You should always take at least five minutes to stretch after you finish your training session. A post-workout stretch promotes strength and flexibility, and helps prevent the *Delayed Onset Muscle Soreness* (DOMS) that can occur the day after you engage in vigorous exercise. By reducing muscle tension and promoting relaxation, stretching enhances the quality of your muscular recovery. In addition, consistent stretching helps prevent injuries by allowing for freer, more integrated movements.

Stretching should never involve sharp, jerky movements or "cheating" with momentum. Human tissue resists force when it is applied too rapidly. In addition, a protective reflex causes your muscles to contract when your tendons sense a fast length change. Your muscles will also contract in response to pain. Obviously, it's impossible to achieve a full stretch with contracted muscles! Always move gradu-ally into the stretched position and stop at the point of mild discomfort, not out-right pain.

Stretching should be just as much a part of your regular work out routine as the exercises themselves. The following is a simple stretching routine that will take no more than five minutes to complete. On pages 150–156, you will find an illustrated explanation of each movement. For best results, do these stretches re-ligiously after every workout.

1. frog-legs (adductor stretch)

2. pie-bows (hamstring stretch)

3. tush-twists (glute stretch)

4. pelicans (quadriceps stretch)

5. rag-dolls (spine stretch)

6. strippers (biceps/chest stretch)

7. towel-tugs (triceps/shoulder stretch)

Step 5: Maximize Your Between-Workout Recovery

Even if you are currently active, the first time you do the Phase 1 exercise rou-tine, your muscles will probably feel a little stiff and sore for a day or two. Rest assured, you will not experience soreness every time you work out. In the vast realm of exercise, pain is not a prerequisite for progress; the old adage "no pain, no gain" is pure nonsense.

It's normal to feel somewhat stiff and sore after challenging your muscles with novel movements. By your third or fourth training session, you should no longer experience muscle soreness the day after your workout. In the meantime, take it easy while your body acclimates to the routine. If you're sore after your first couple of exercise sessions, the judicious use of over-the-counter nonsteroidal anti-inflammatory drugs (NSAIDs) like Aspirin or ibuprofen can provide relief. During the initial week of training, I also recommend repeating your post-workout stretches before you go to bed every night.

Step 6: Smile. Your new look is just weeks away!

Step-ups

1. STEP-UPS are a great, nonimpact way to continue warming up. Step-ups will gradually raise both core temperature and heart rate to the metabolism-revving anaerobic zone.

TARGET MUSCLES: glutes, hamstrings, and quadriceps.

AESTHETIC AND HEALTH BENEFITS: overall fat burning, butt lifting, and thigh trimming.

FUNCTIONAL AND ATHLETIC BENEFITS: improved balance, increased leg strength and stamina.

EQUIPMENT REQUIRED: a stable, raised surface such as a step, or a sturdy coffee table.

HOW TO DO IT: Start with your feet together. Step onto the raised surface one foot at a time. Step back down to the floor one foot at a time. Do this 20 times, leading with the same foot (right or left), then repeat the sequence starting with the opposite foot for 20 additional repetitions.

WHAT **NOT** TO DO: Never use a step height that exceeds your knee height.

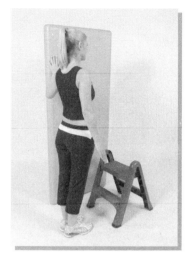

1

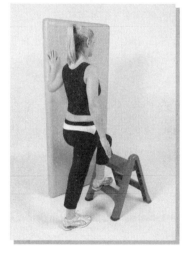

2

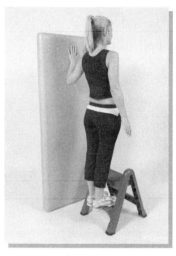

3

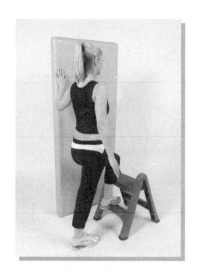

4

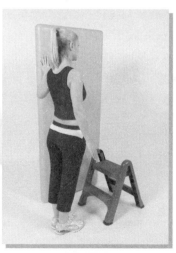

5

121

Push-ups

2. PUSH-UPS permit your heart rate to recover to the fat-burning aerobic zone while you strengthen your deltoids, pectorals, and triceps. The multijoint nature of this exercise warms your upper body and prepares it for the remainder of the workout. Depending on your fitness level, there are two different levels of difficulty to choose from when doing push-ups.

TARGET MUSCLES: core muscles, pectorals, triceps, and deltoids.

AESTHETIC AND HEALTH BENEFITS: strong pectorals boost your bust while toned triceps help eradicate upper arm jiggle. Shapely shoulders confer a more confident bearing.

FUNCTIONAL AND ATHLETIC BENEFITS: increased upper body strength, stamina, and coordination.

NOVICE PUSH-UPS

EQUIPMENT REQUIRED: a stable surface of less than waist height. I recommend using the arm of a sofa, the edge of a heavy coffee table, or a workout bench.

HOW TO DO IT: Place your hands in front of you, about shoulder width apart, on the stable surface. Then, supporting your weight with your outstretched arms, walk backwards until your waist is straight. This is your starting position. From here, slowly bend your elbows and lower your chest toward the stable surface. When your elbows form right angles, stop your descent and begin extending your arms to push your body back up to the starting position. Once you are able to complete 20 repetitions of novice push-ups, advance to regular push-ups for your next workout.

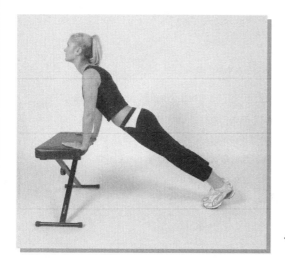

1

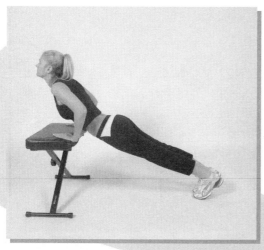

2

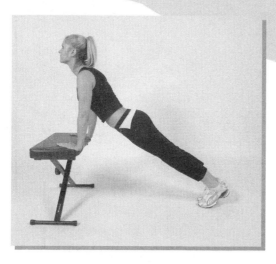

3

WHAT **NOT** TO DO: Don't bend at the waist; keep your back, butt, and legs straight throughout the movement.

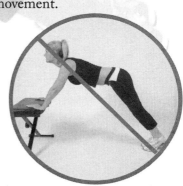

REGULAR PUSH-UPS

EQUIPMENT REQUIRED: a clean floor or workout mat.

HOW TO DO IT: Keeping your arms straight, place your hands about shoulder width apart on the floor or workout mat. Supporting your weight with your outstretched arms, walk backward until your waist is straight. This is your starting position. From here, slowly bend your arms and lower your chest toward the floor. When your arms form right angles at the elbow, stop your descent and push your body back up to the starting position. Repeat up to 30 times.

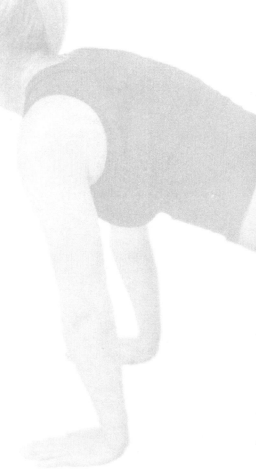

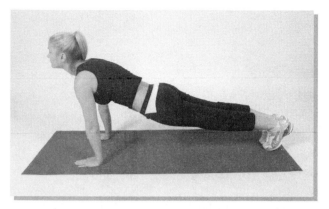

1

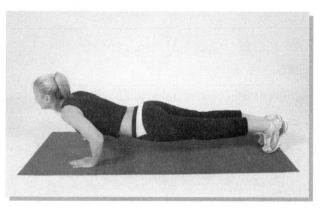

2

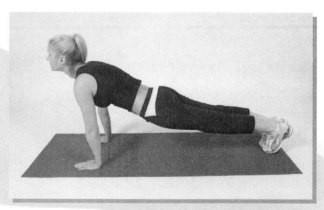

3

WHAT **NOT** TO DO: Don't bend at the waist; keep your back, butt, and legs straight throughout the movement.

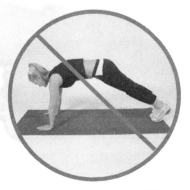

Lunge-curls

3. LUNGE-CURLS are multijoint exercises involving both your lower and upper body. These movements act to rapidly reaccelerate your heart rate right back to the metabolism-elevating anaerobic zone.

TARGET MUSCLES: core muscles, glutes, hamstrings, quadriceps, and biceps.

AESTHETIC AND HEALTH BENEFITS: overall fat burning, butt lifting, and thigh trimming. Bicep curls will tighten and define your upper arms.

FUNCTIONAL AND ATHLETIC BENEFITS: improved balance and coordination, increased arm and leg strength.

EQUIPMENT REQUIRED: two soup cans or a pair of light dumbbells.

HOW TO DO IT: Start with your feet together and arms at your sides. Hold a light dumbbell in each hand. This is your starting position. From here, step forward (with your choice of leading foot) and lower yourself into a lunged position. As your leading foot comes forward, curl both dumbbells toward your shoulders by simultaneously flexing both elbows. As you step back to the starting position, lower both dumbbells back to your sides. Alternate leading legs as you repeat this exercise for up to 20 repetitions per leg.

WHAT **NOT** TO DO: Never flex your leading leg beyond 90 degrees at the knee.

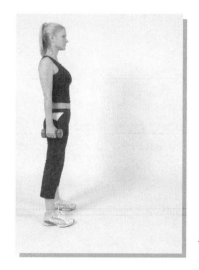 1

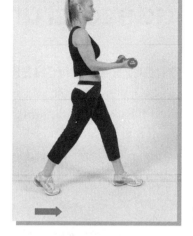 2

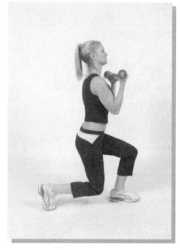 3

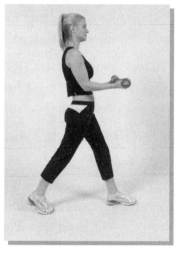 4

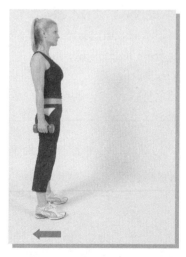 5

Squeeze-crunches

4. SQUEEZE-CRUNCHES allow your heart rate to recover to the fat-burning aerobic zone while you target your abdominal musculature. Squeeze-crunches differ from conventional crunches by virtue of a sustained hamstring contraction that acts to disengage the hip flexors. As a result, all the crunch motion derives solely from the rectus abdominus or "six-pack" muscles. Squeeze-crunches are the most efficient way to work your abs without special equipment.

TARGET MUSCLES: rectus abdominus, hamstrings, and glutes.

AESTHETIC AND HEALTH BENEFITS: strong abs and a flat stomach don't just look good, they also help to stabilize your core musculature, improve your posture, eliminate low back pain, and prevent future back injury.

FUNCTIONAL AND ATHLETIC BENEFITS: a stronger core increases overall coordination. The sustained hamstring squeeze increases hamstring stamina and tightens your tush.

EQUIPMENT REQUIRED: a cushion or athletic ball (soccer ball, volleyball, or basketball), and an exercise mat or carpeted area.

HOW TO DO IT: Start by lying on your back. Bend your knees toward your chest and squeeze the cushion or athletic ball between the back of your thighs and the back of your lower legs. Place your hands by your ears with your elbows pointed out. This is your starting position. Continue to squeeze the cushion or ball behind your knees as you exhale and "crunch" your abdominal muscles, moving your nose toward your knees. Your shoulder blades should leave the floor but your neck should not flex. Hold the contraction for a half count, then inhale as you return to the starting position. Repeat up to 30 times.

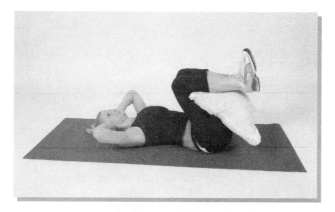

1

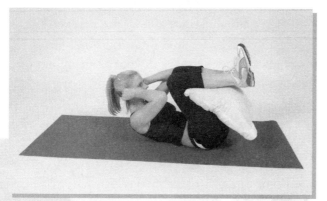

2

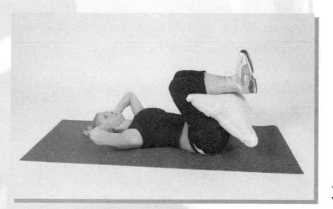

3

WHAT **NOT** TO DO: Don't grab the back of your head or neck with your hands. Doing so will tempt you to torque your chin toward your chest during the crunch motion, which does nothing for your abs but can strain your neck muscles.

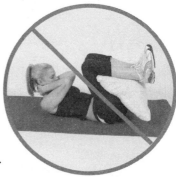

Squat-presses

5. SQUAT-PRESSES combine the butt-blasting power of a wide-stance squat with an overhead shoulder movement. The complex, multijoint nature of this exercise acts to reaccelerate your heart rate back into the metabolism-revving anaerobic zone.

TARGET MUSCLES: core muscles, glutes, hamstrings, quads, and deltoids.

AESTHETIC AND HEALTH BENEFITS: wide squats are one of the best ways to target the entire gluteal complex and thighs for overall fat burning, butt lifting, and thigh toning. The overhead press increases shoulder and upper back definition.

FUNCTIONAL AND ATHLETIC BENEFITS: wide squats increase explosive leg strength, while overhead presses build shoulder strength in a motion range where many individuals (women in particular) are extremely lacking.

EQUIPMENT REQUIRED: two soup cans or a pair of light dumbbells.

HOW TO DO IT: Hold the light dumbbells at shoulder height. Stand with your feet about twice shoulder width apart. Keep your chin up and your back straight as you squat down until your thighs are nearly parallel to the floor. This is your starting position. From the squatted position, push through your heels and lift the light dumbbells straight up over your head as you rise back to the standing position. Repeat up to 30 times.

WHAT NOT TO DO: Low squats place unnecessary strain on your patellar tendons and knee joints. Never squat to the point that your thighs descend below parallel to the floor.

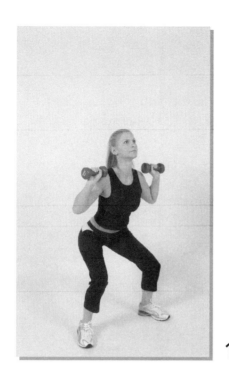

1

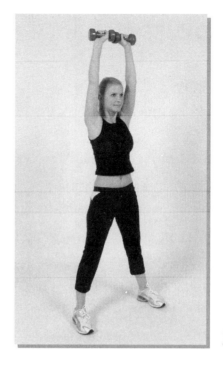

2

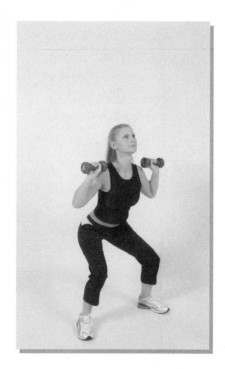

3

Rows

6. ROWS are a straightforward movement that targets both back and arm musculature while permitting heart rate deceleration to the fat-burning aerobic zone.

TARGET MUSCLES: spinal erectors, latissimus dorsi, and biceps.

AESTHETIC AND HEALTH BENEFITS: rows are a great movement for improving posture and adding definition to your back and arms.

FUNCTIONAL AND ATHLETIC BENEFITS: increases overall upper body strength and stamina.

EQUIPMENT REQUIRED: two soup cans or a pair of light dumbbells and a stable, horizontal surface like a door or wall.

HOW TO DO IT: Hold a light dumbbell in each hand as you position yourself so that you are standing about a foot from a stable, vertical surface, facing out. Plant your feet approximately shoulder width apart and bend at the knees and waist so that your torso forms a more or less right angle with your thighs, and your butt is pressed against the horizontal surface for support. This is your starting position. From here, keep your back straight, head up, and elbows close to your sides as you pull the dumbbells straight up until they contact your torso. At this point, your elbows should actually be pointing slightly above your torso. Pause for a moment before lowering the dumbbells back to the starting position. Repeat up to 30 times.

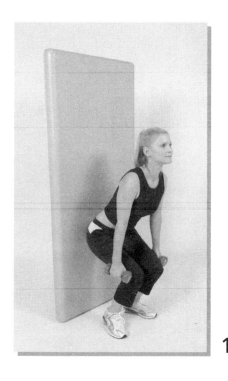

1

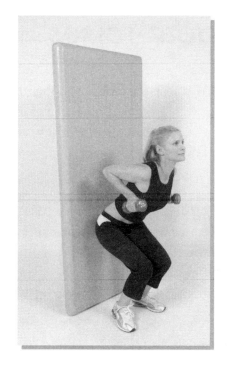

2

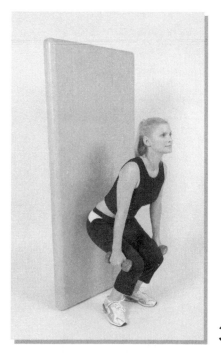

3

WHAT **NOT** TO DO: Do not relax your spine, slouch, or slump forward at any point during the movement.

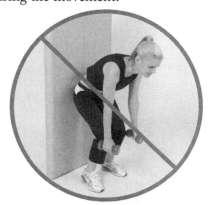

Squat-raises

7. SQUAT-RAISES combine the thigh-toning power of a narrow-stance squat with a lateral shoulder movement. Like its cousin the squat-press, the complex, multijoint nature of this exercise acts to reaccelerate heart rate to the metabolism-revving anaerobic zone.

TARGET MUSCLES: core muscles, quads, glutes, hamstrings, and deltoids.

AESTHETIC AND HEALTH BENEFITS: narrow squats are one of the best ways to induce overall fat burning while toning and defining your thighs. Squat-raises also target glutes and hamstrings. Lateral raises increase shoulder definition.

FUNCTIONAL AND ATHLETIC BENEFITS: narrow squats increase quad strength and stamina while lateral raises build shoulder strength.

EQUIPMENT REQUIRED: two soup cans or a pair of light dumbbells.

HOW TO DO IT: Hold the light dumbbells at your side while you stand with your feet about shoulder width apart. Keep your chin up and your back straight as you squat down until your thighs are nearly parallel to the floor. From the squatted position, push from the balls of your feet and raise the light dumbbells out to your sides until they are parallel to your shoulders as you rise back to the standing position. Repeat up to 30 times.

WHAT NOT TO DO: Low squats place unnecessary strain on your patellar tendons and knee joints. Never squat to the point that your thighs descend below parallel to the floor.

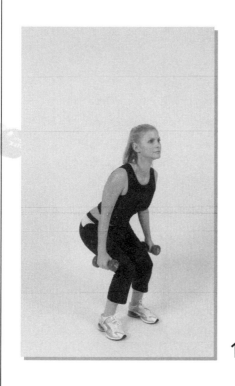

1

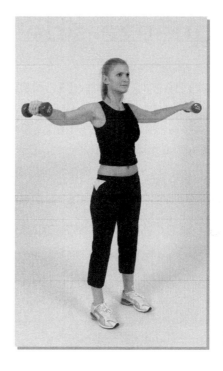

2

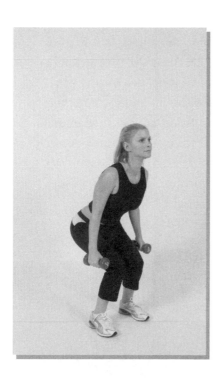

3

Squeeze-side-crunch

8. SQUEEZE-SIDE-CRUNCHES allow your heart rate to recover to the fat-burning aerobic zone while targeting the oblique and rectus abdominus musculature. Like standard squeeze-crunches, squeeze-side-crunches require a sustained hamstring contraction that acts to disengage the hip flexors. As a result, the crunch motion specifically targets the oblique and rectus muscles.

TARGET MUSCLES: obliques, rectus abdominus, and hamstrings.

AESTHETIC AND HEALTH BENEFITS: strong obliques help to stabilize core musculature during torso rotation.

FUNCTIONAL AND ATHLETIC BENEFITS: a stronger core increases overall coordination, improves posture, helps to eradicate low back pain, and can prevent future back injury. The sustained hamstring squeeze increases hamstring stamina and tightens your tush.

EQUIPMENT REQUIRED: pillow or athletic ball (soccer ball, volleyball, or basketball), and exercise mat or carpeted area.

HOW TO DO IT: Start by lying on your back. Bend your knees toward your chest and squeeze the pillow or athletic ball between the back of your thighs and the back of your lower legs. Place your hands by your ears with your elbows pointed out. This is your starting position. Continue to squeeze the pillow or ball behind your knees as you exhale and "crunch" your abdominal muscles, moving your right elbow toward your left knee. Your right shoulder blade should leave the floor but your neck should not flex. Hold the contraction for a half count, then return to the starting position. Repeat on the opposite side, bringing your left elbow toward your right knee. Do up to 15 repetitions per side for a total of 30 repetitions.

WHAT NOT TO DO: As with regular squeeze-crunches, you should never grab the back of your head or neck with your hands.

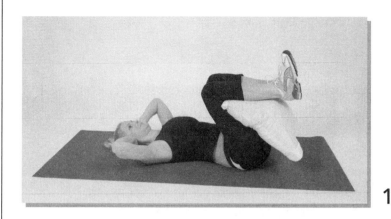

1

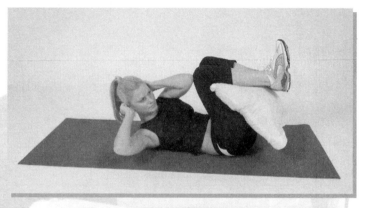

2

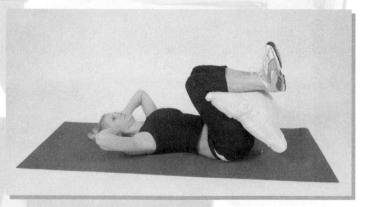

3

137

Sissy-squats

9. SISSY-SQUATS mark the beginning of the cool down phase of the workout. While maintaining heart rate in the fat-burning aerobic zone, the *isometric contraction* (iso = same; metric = length) at the peak of the sissy-squat builds lactate threshold and local endurance. Sissy-squats might seem easy at first, but you will feel the burn by the end of the set. Depending on your fitness level and easy access to a stair railing or sturdy door handle, there are two different levels of difficulty to choose from when doing sissy-squats.

TARGET MUSCLES: glutes and quads.

AESTHETIC AND HEALTH BENEFITS: sissy-squats are the perfect finishing exercise for fatigued glutes and quads. Sissy-squats help define and tone the thighs while lifting the butt from yet another angle.

FUNCTIONAL AND ATHLETIC BENEFITS: increased lactate threshold translates to increased lower body stamina.

NOVICE SISSY-SQUATS

HOW TO DO IT: Place your hands on your hips and plant your feet firmly on the floor about shoulder width apart. Keeping your head up and your back straight, lower your butt toward the floor. Descend as low as your strength and flexibility allow. For sissy-squats, it is safe to descend below a 90 degree angle at the knee and let your heels come off the floor. Pause for a moment in the fully squatted position and concentrate on tightening your butt as you begin to ascend. At the peak of the motion when you're fully upright, thrust your pelvis forward and squeeze your butt cheeks for a full count (one-Mississippi) before executing the next repetition. Repeat up to 20 times. Once you are able to complete 20 repetitions of novice sissy-squats, advance to regular sissy-squats for your next workout.

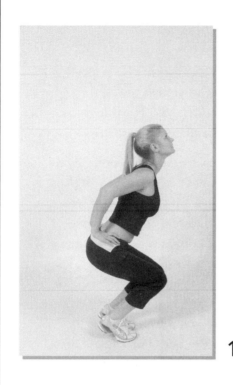

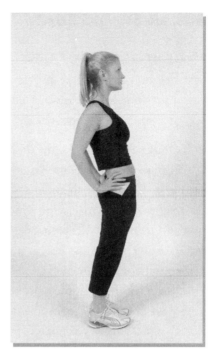

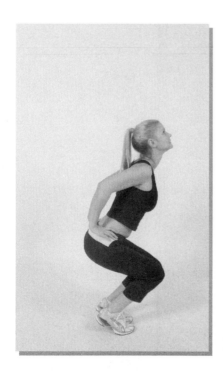

1

3

2

REGULAR SISSY-SQUATS

EQUIPMENT REQUIRED: A fixed, sturdy item that can either be gripped at waist height, or that you can pass a short length of rope (or a towel) through to support your weight at waist height. A stair banister, balcony railing, squat rack, or even a door knob in a heavy-duty door are all good alternatives.

HOW TO DO IT: Grasp the fixed object (or rope/towel ends) with both hands and drop an imaginary line straight down to the floor between your wrists. Place your feet about shoulder width apart on either side of the point where the imaginary line meets the ground. Grasping the rope ends, extend your arms and lean back. Keep your legs, waist, and back straight as you assume a "water-skiing" position. This is your starting point. Keeping your back and arms straight, squat down to the point that your butt nearly contacts the floor. Pause for a moment in the fully squatted position and concentrate on tightening your butt as you begin to ascend. At the peak of the motion when you're fully upright, thrust your pelvis forward and squeeze your butt cheeks for a full count (one-Mississippi) before executing the next repetition. Repeat up to 30 times.

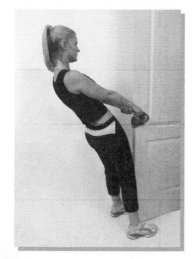

1

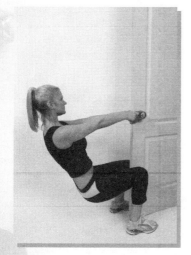

2

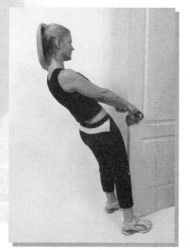

3

Bench-dips

10. BENCH-DIPS are the ultimate triceps challenge and are guaranteed to maintain an elevated heart rate for continued fat burning. Depending on your current fitness level, you can choose from three different levels of difficulty when doing this exercise: novice, regular, or advanced bench-dips.

TARGET MUSCLES: triceps, deltoids, and pectorals.

AESTHETIC AND HEALTH BENEFITS: bench dips eradicate upper arm jiggle.

FUNCTIONAL AND ATHLETIC BENEFITS: increased upper body strength, stamina, and coordination.

EQUIPMENT REQUIRED: stable surface of less than waist height. I recommend using the arm of a sofa, the edge of a heavy coffee table, or a workout bench.

NOVICE BENCH-DIPS

HOW TO DO IT: To begin, sit on the edge of the stable surface with your hands on either side of your butt. Hold your torso upright with your fully extended arms and keep your knees bent as you slide your butt off the front of the stable surface. This is your starting position. Flex your elbows and knees as you lower your butt towards the floor. Descend until your upper arms are roughly parallel to the floor. At this point, stop your descent and push your body back up to the starting position. Use as much arm strength with as little help from your legs as possible. Once you are able to complete 20 repetitions of novice bench-dips, advance to regular bench-dips for your next workout.

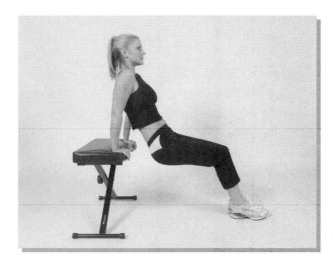

1

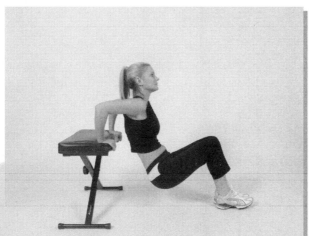

2

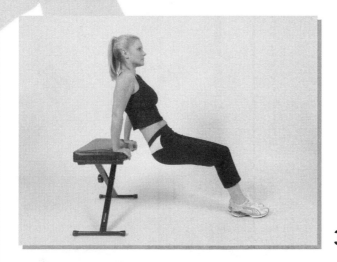

3

143

REGULAR BENCH-DIPS

HOW TO DO IT: To begin, sit on the edge of the stable surface with your hands on either side of your butt. Hold your torso upright with your fully extended arms and slide your butt off the front of the stable surface. Extend your legs out in front of you until your knees are straight. This is your starting position. Flex your elbows as you lower your butt towards the floor. Descend until your upper arms are roughly parallel to the floor. At this point, stop your descent and push your body back up to the starting position. Repeat up to 20 times. Once you are able to complete 20 repetitions of regular bench-dips, progress to advanced bench dips for your next workout.

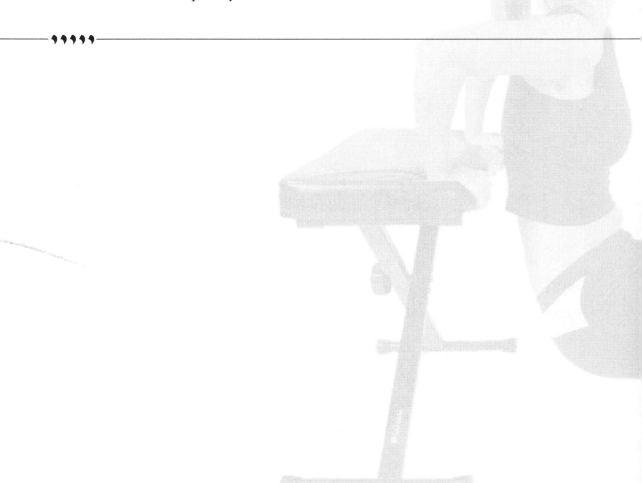

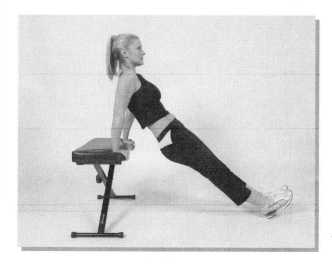

1

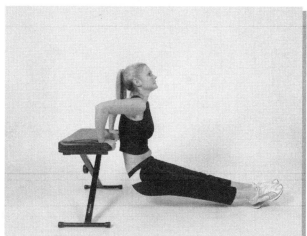

2

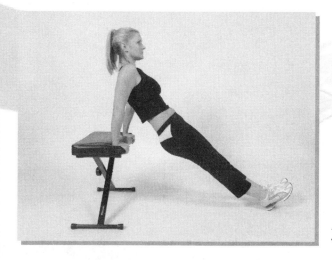

3

145

ADVANCED BENCH-DIPS

HOW TO DO IT: Begin by placing a second stable surface opposite the first. The distance between them should be roughly the length of your legs. To begin, sit on the edge of the stable surface with your hands on either side of your butt. Holding your torso upright with your fully extended arms, slide your butt off the front of the stable surface, place your feet onto the opposite surface, and extend your legs so that your knees are straight. This is your starting position. Flex your elbows as you lower your butt towards the floor. Descend until your upper arms are roughly parallel to the floor. At this point, stop your descent and push your body back up to the starting position. Repeat up to 30 times.

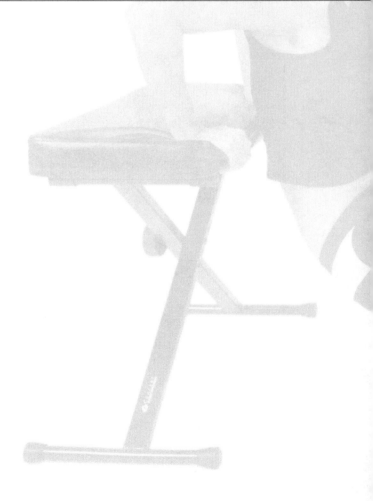

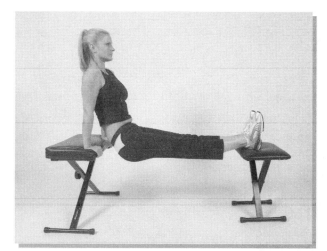

1

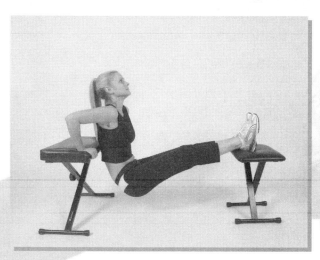

2

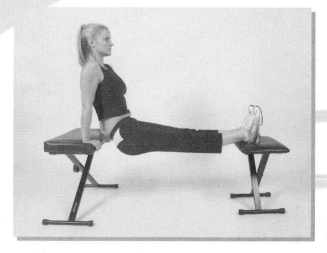

3

147

Calf-raises

11. CALF-RAISES target your calves while allowing for gradual heart rate deceleration. The combination of *concentric* (when the muscle is in the process of flexing) and *isometric* (when the muscle is holding a flexed or partly flexed position) contractions builds both strength and local endurance. Like sissy-squats, calf-raises are a great finishing exercise for fatigued muscles.

TARGET MUSCLES: gastrocnemius and soleus muscles.

AESTHETIC AND HEALTH BENEFITS: toned, defined calves.

FUNCTIONAL AND ATHLETIC BENEFITS: improved balance, enhanced ankle stability, and increased lower leg strength and stamina.

EQUIPMENT REQUIRED: a stable, raised surface such as a step.

HOW TO DO IT: Stand with your toes on the edge of the step. Lower your heels below the step as far as your balance and flexibility allow. This is your starting position. From here, extend your calves (by rising up on your toes) as high as you can. Squeeze your calves for a half-count at the peak of the motion, then slowly return to the starting position and repeat up to 30 times.

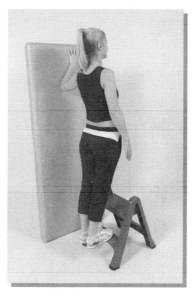

1

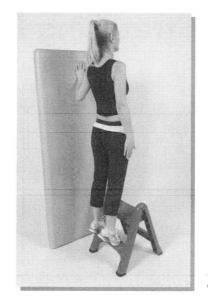

2

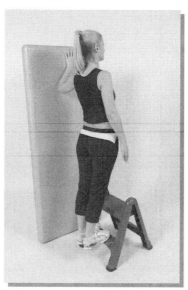

3

12. A final set of **SQUEEZE-CRUNCHES** completes the routine.

The Stretching Routine

GENERAL INSTRUCTIONS FOR EFFECTIVE STRETCHING: Stretch within the safe limits of your flexibility by moving slowly into the stretched position and stopping when you reach the point of mild discomfort. Exhale and hold the full stretch for 20 seconds, then breath deeply as you release. Do each stretch twice before moving onto the next.

Frog-legs

1. FROG-LEGS are a great way to stretch the adductor muscles of your inner thighs. Sit on the floor with your knees bent and your feet touching. Keeping your feet together, slowly push your knees down toward the floor on either side. Hold the stretch for 20 seconds, relax, and repeat.

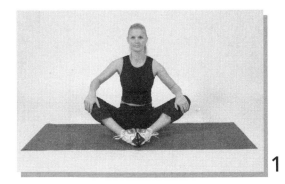 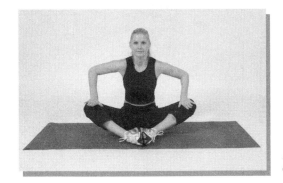

1

2

Pie-bows

2. PIE-BOWS target your hamstrings. Start by sitting on the floor with your legs straight out and spread as far apart as your flexibility permits. Keeping your back as straight as possible, reach for your left foot as you bend at the waist and lower your chin over your left knee. Hold the stretch for 20 seconds, relax, and repeat. Repeat the entire sequence over your right knee. Then repeat the sequence between your legs, lowering your chin toward the floor.

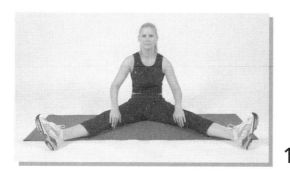

1

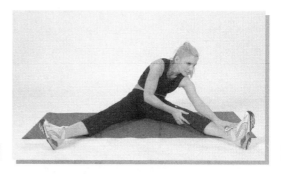

2

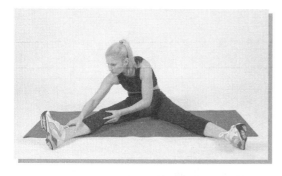

3

4

Tush-twists

3. TUSH-TWISTS target your glutes and spine. Start by sitting on the floor with both legs straight out in front of you. Support yourself with your right hand as you cross your right foot over your left knee. Then push against your right knee with your left elbow as you turn your torso clockwise to look back over your right shoulder. Hold for 20 seconds, relax, and repeat. Repeat the entire sequence on your opposite side.

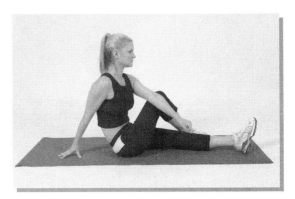

1

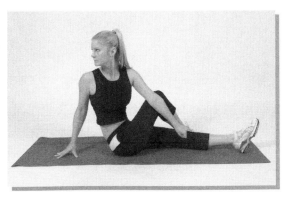

2

Pelicans

4. PELICANS are a simple, effective stretch for your quadriceps. If necessary, feel free to use a chair or table to steady yourself. From a standing position, lift your right foot back toward your butt and grab your right ankle with your right hand. While firmly holding your ankle, push your bent knee down until it is perpendicular to the floor. Hold for 20 seconds, relax, and repeat. Repeat the entire sequence with your left leg.

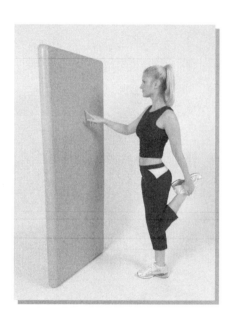

Rag-dolls

5. RAG-DOLLS are a painless way to stretch your neck and back. Stand with your feet no more than shoulder width apart. Keep your legs straight, but don't lock your knees. Starting at the base of your skull, relax the muscles that support your spine from top to bottom. Let your head loll forward, followed by your shoulders, upper back, and then the rest of your torso. Hang for 20 seconds, straighten, and repeat.

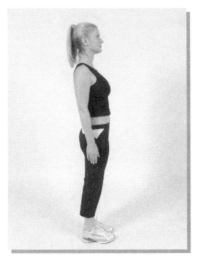

1

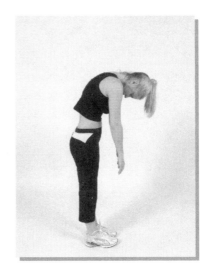

2

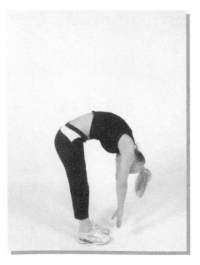

3

Strippers

6. STRIPPERS are a great stretch for your biceps, chest, and shoulders. You will need a stable surface at approximately shoulder height. If there are no fire poles available, a door jamb is a good substitute. Raise your right arm to shoulder height. Keeping your elbow straight, press your right palm against the surface. Now, slowly turn your head and torso counterclockwise and away from your right shoulder. Hold for 20 seconds, relax, and repeat. Repeat the entire sequence using your left arm.

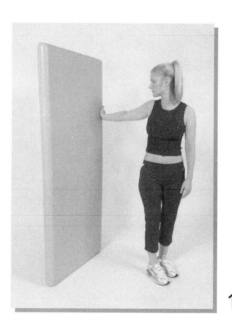
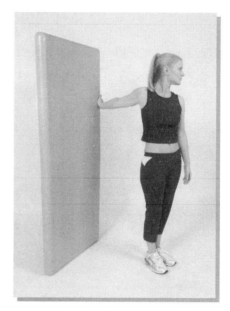

Towel-tugs

7. TOWEL-TUGS stretch your triceps and shoulders like no other stretch can. You will need either a hand towel or a short length of rope to do them properly. Start by standing with your feet about shoulder width apart. Grip the towel in your right hand and flip it over your shoulder. Grab the other end of the towel behind your back with your left hand. Point your right elbow toward the ceiling and pull gently on the towel with your left hand to provide a downward counterforce and increase the range of the stretch. Hold for 20 seconds, relax, and repeat. Repeat the entire sequence with your opposite side.

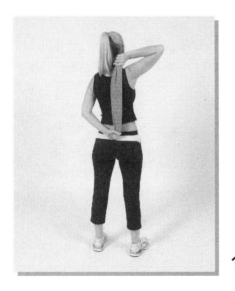

1

2

THE PHASE 2 WORKOUT (WEEKS 4–6)

By the beginning of week 4, the fatigue you may have experienced during the first week is a distant memory. Indeed, you are now sleeping more soundly and feeling more refreshed and energetic than you have in years. Your skin is starting to glow and your hair is becoming increasingly luminous. Your arms and shoulders have new definition, and you've lost inches across your back and midriff. As love handles and belly bulge begin to melt away, the underlying musculature tightens, flattening your abs, straightening your spine, and pulling your shoulders back. And as your posture improves, your bearing appears taller, stronger, and more confident.

And your pants are fitting differently! Saddle bags and thigh jiggle are disappearing. Your legs are gaining definition and your butt is lifting. Once you are within five to ten pounds of your ideal body weight, don't be surprised if the lifting and tightening of your glutes and hamstrings minimizes the apparent changes in your lower body measurements. As body fat is dispatched, the resulting volume loss may approximate the volume gain caused by the elevation of your posterior contours. Don't despair; the simultaneous muscle toning and fat burning equates to a smoother, firmer, and perkier topography.

Phase 2 continues fostering improvements in body composition as your fabulous physique takes shape. You have now created a muscle base and increased growth hormone production. In addition, your new eating habits and supplementation regimen have gone a long way toward reestablishing a healthy physiological equilibrium and stable homeostasis. Put simply, your body is beginning to run like the brilliantly assembled, well-oiled machine it was designed to be. *You are now primed for physical metamorphosis!* From this point forward, your physique will literally transform before your eyes as every passing week brings visible, tangible improvements.

By now, along with increased muscle tone, a leaner body composition, and a revved metabolism, you've also gained new strength, stamina, and coordination. You are probably finding that the 20-minute Phase 1 routine has become progressively less challenging. You may even be completing the workout in under 20 minutes. It's time to take it up a notch! With your improved fitness level, you are ready to add some new exercises. But don't worry—the Phase 2 workout routine should only take about 25 minutes to complete. In fact, the only difference between the Phase 1 routine and the Phase 2 routine is one additional quartet. Instead of completing *three* quartets (12 sets of exercises) for a workout duration of about 20 minutes, you will now complete *four* quartets (16 sets) for a workout duration of about 25 minutes.

PHASE 2 WORKOUT SCHEDULE

For the next three weeks, the Phase 2 routine should be completed using the four on/one off schedule you implemented for weeks 2 and 3 of Phase 1. *(The compliance forms for weeks 4–6 in Appendix C list the appropriate exercise routine with rest days indicated.)* As always, take three to five minutes before you begin your workout to warm up, and at least five minutes to stretch after you finish your training session.

New Exercises

The expanded routine includes two new movements, **horse curls** and **wide sissy-squats**. Both are illustrated and explained on pages 160–163.

CONTINUED PROGRESS

The *Ten Years Thinner* program was created to yield lifelong results. Once you have attained the physique of your dreams, it is relatively simple to maintain your new look. (This will be explained in more detail in Chapter 10.) However, in order to continue making rapid progress during Phase 2 and beyond, your training intensity must increase at roughly the same rate as your conditioning. Fortunately, there is a very simple way to ensure that you are exercising at a level that is sufficiently challenging. As was already discussed briefly, the number of recommended repetitions per set is a basic guideline. If and when your strength and stamina increase to the point that you can easily do additional repetitions, then it's time to raise the height of the step, move on to a more advanced version of the exercise, or increase the denomination of your weights by a pound or two.

The vast majority of *Ten Years Thinner* program participants were thrilled with the progress they observed using the basic 25-minute exercise routine. However, a small portion of my test subjects (less than 5 percent) wanted more. For these go-getters, I designed a 30-minute routine with one additional quartet for a total of 20 exercise sets. But before we move on to that, I'd like to emphasize that the 30-minute routine is *entirely optional!* You will enjoy great results with the basic, 25-minute Phase 2 routine.

OPTIONAL 30-MINUTE WORKOUT SCHEDULE

Just like the basic Phase 2 routine, the optional 30-minute routine should be completed using a four on one off schedule. As always, take three to five minutes before you begin your workout to warm up, and at least five minutes to stretch after you finish your training session.

New Exercises

The optional 30-minute routine includes two new movements, *reverse lunge-front-raises* and a vestige of PE commonly referred to as *squat-thrusts*. See pages 164–167.

Horse Curls

HORSE CURLS combine the toning power of a sustained squat with a compound upper-body movement that targets both arms and shoulders. This exercise accelerates your heart rate into the anaerobic zone.

TARGET MUSCLES: glutes, hamstrings, quads, biceps, and deltoids.

AESTHETIC AND HEALTH BENEFITS: The *isometric* (see below) nature of this exercise increases thigh definition while toning your tush. The combined bicep curl/shoulder press contributes to arm, shoulder, and upper back definition.

FUNCTIONAL AND ATHLETIC BENEFITS: This exercise helps build lower body stamina, upper body strength, and overall balance.

EQUIPMENT REQUIRED: two soup cans or a pair of light dumbbells.

HOW TO DO IT: If you have ever studied martial arts, you are probably already familiar with the *horse stance*. In essence, you place your feet about double shoulder width apart and lower your butt straight down toward the floor as if you intend to do a wide squat. However, rather than sinking all the way to the point where your thighs are parallel to the floor (as you would do for a wide squat), end your descent once your knees form right angles. You will hold this position for the duration of the exercise. Because your lower body doesn't move, the muscles holding you steady (mostly your quads, hamstrings, and glutes) are in a constant state of isometric contraction.

The upper body component of horse curls is a multijoint movement that starts with a bicep curl and progresses to an overhead shoulder press. Begin by holding the dumbbells down at your sides as you assume horse stance. Then, flex both elbows simultaneously, bringing the weights toward your shoulders so that your palms are facing you at the top of the bicep curl. Transition smoothly from the top of the bicep curl into a shoulder press. Remember to rotate your wrists out as you push the dumbbells straight overhead. Once your arms are fully extended at the top of the shoulder press, your palms should be facing away from you. Do the exact reverse as you lower your arms back to their starting positions at your sides.

While your lower body remains in horse stance, repeat the curl-presses for between 20 and 30 repetitions.

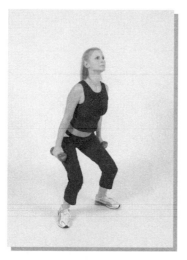

1

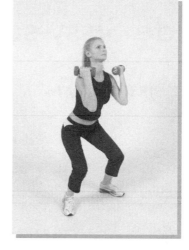

2

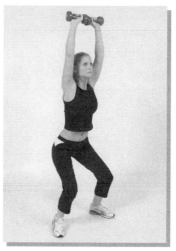

3

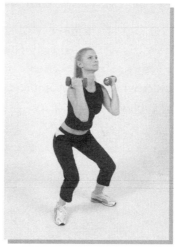

4

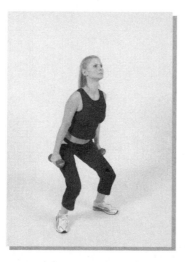

5

WHAT NOT TO DO: Don't get discouraged if you are unable to complete the recommended 20 to 30 curl-presses while maintaining your lower body in horse stance. Almost no one (myself included!) does this exercise all the way through the first time they try. Rather than giving up once your lower body fatigues, straighten your legs for two or three curl-presses and then sink back down into horse stance to complete your set.

Wide Sissy-squats

WIDE SISSY-SQUATS can be completed in either the novice or regular sissy-squat stances.

TARGET MUSCLES: glutes and quads.

AESTHETIC AND HEALTH BENEFITS: Like standard sissy-squats, wide sissy-squats help define and tone the thighs, especially the inner thighs, while targeting the butt from yet another angle.

FUNCTIONAL AND ATHLETIC BENEFITS: increased lactate threshold translates to increased lower body stamina.

HOW TO DO IT: Wide sissy squats are nearly identical to the standard version with which you are already familiar, the only difference being the width of your stance. Rather than performing the exercise with your feet positioned shoulder width apart, complete the movements with your feet approximately twice shoulder width apart.

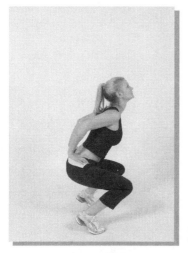

1

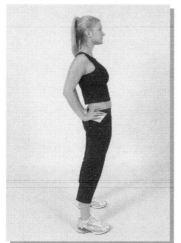

2

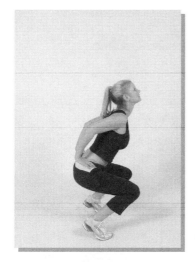

3

Reverse Lunge-front-raises

REVERSE LUNGE-FRONT-RAISES. Like their first cousin, lunge-curls, reverse lunge-front-raises are multijoint exercises, involving both your lower and upper body, that rapidly accelerate your heart rate to the anaerobic zone.

TARGET MUSCLES: core muscles, glutes, hamstrings, quadriceps, and the anterior (front) head of the deltoids.

AESTHETIC AND HEALTH BENEFITS: overall fat burning, butt lifting, and thigh trimming. Front raises will tone and define the front of your shoulders.

FUNCTIONAL AND ATHLETIC BENEFITS: improved balance and coordination, increased shoulder and leg strength.

EQUIPMENT REQUIRED: two soup cans or a pair of light dumbbells.

HOW TO DO IT: Start with your feet together and arms at your sides. Hold a light dumbbell in each hand. From this starting position, step backward with your choice of foot and lower yourself into a lunged position. As your initiating foot travels backward, keep your arms straight as you raise **both** dumbbells out in front of you to shoulder height. As you resume the starting position, lower both dumbbells back to your sides. Alternate legs as you repeat this exercise for up to 20 repetitions per leg.

WHAT NOT TO DO: Never flex your leading leg (the one that stays in front) beyond 90 degrees at the knee.

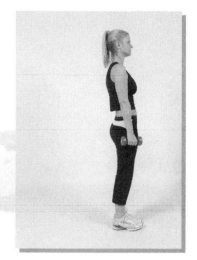

1

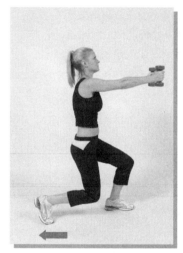

2

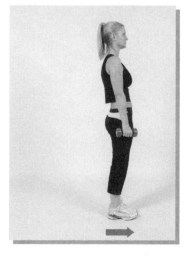

3

165

Squat-thrusts

SQUAT-THRUSTS build power and agility while spiking your heart rate back into the anaerobic zone. This calisthenic movement should be done rapidly.

TARGET MUSCLES: core muscles, glutes, hamstrings, and quadriceps.

AESTHETIC AND HEALTH BENEFITS: lower-body toning.

FUNCTIONAL AND ATHLETIC BENEFITS: increased power and agility.

EQUIPMENT REQUIRED: a clean floor or exercise mat.

HOW TO DO IT: Start by standing tall with your arms down at your sides. Bend your knees and drop onto all fours. Then, with your hands planted firmly on the floor, jump-thrust your legs straight out behind you into push-up position. From there, jump-pull your legs back to the squatted position and stand, resuming the start position. Repeat 30 times.

WHAT NOT TO DO: Don't let unpleasant memories of gym class distract you from using good form.

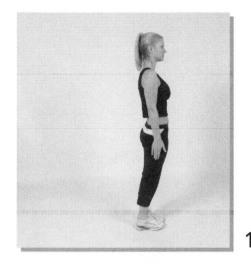

1

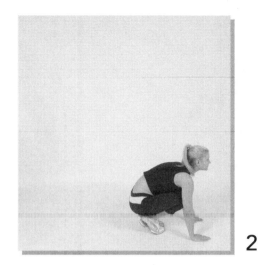

2

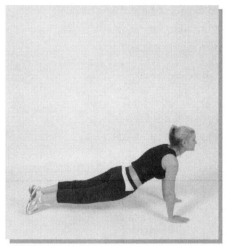

3

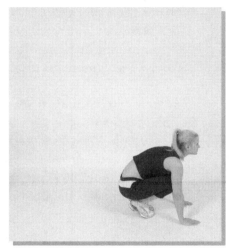

4

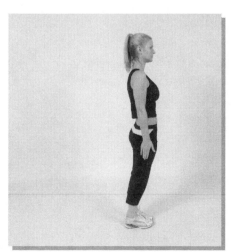

5

———— ♦♦♦♦♦ ————

"I can't thank Dr. Lydon enough for introducing
me to this program. It's been over a year and I'm still
on track and feeling great!" — DARLENE, 43

"People are always worried about how they're going to
stick to their diet when they leave their home environment.
But with *Ten Years Thinner*, whether you go to a
restaurant or a friend's house for dinner, it's easy to
follow the guidelines just about anywhere." — JILLIAN, 38

"I think a lot of diets have come apart with one bad meal.
People get so wracked with guilt over one transgression that
they give up. With *Ten Years Thinner*, the weekly cheat meal
gives you permission to transgress once in a while
and feel OK about it. It's a very effective way
to help maintain motivation." — MATT, 38

———— ♦♦♦♦♦ ————

CHAPTER ,,, 10

Forever Young

Congratulations! You have been eating right and exercising regularly for several weeks. Whether you've attained your ideal body composition by the end of week 6, or your physique is still a work in progress, you have discovered that a healthy lifestyle is no more time consuming or complicated than the average unhealthy lifestyle. You are living proof that the increased focus and energy that accompany healthy living can make every facet of your life feel easier and more enjoyable.

At the six-week marker, you have toned your muscles, revved your metabolism, and transformed your internal furnace from one that burns sugar to one that burns fat. Thanks to your new eating habits and supplementation regimen, you are on the road to reestablishing the steadfast homeostasis of a time that predated the pro-inflammatory assaults of contemporary living, assaults that have since turned our physiological equilibrium into a precariously balanced mess.

Now for the bad news: If you abandon your new eating and exercise habits, your body, skin, and overall health will gradually begin to backslide. However, you won't start packing on the pounds right away. As I mentioned in Chapter 1, unlike other popular diet plans, the *Ten Years Thinner* program hasn't turned you into a smaller, flabbier, hungrier version of your former self. On the contrary, your energy is probably higher than it's been in years. In fact, you have never been more primed for continued progress.

A Program for Real Life

Four months after embracing the Ten Years Thinner program and losing a combined total of more than 50 pounds, Matt and Jillian Edwards were confronted by circumstances that forced them to take a break from their new healthy lifestyle. They both feared they would immediately start to regain the weight.

"When a family emergency pulled me out of town for three weeks, I ate all my meals at hospital cafeterias, greasy spoons, and other people's houses. Alcohol was served at dinner almost every evening. And I didn't exercise once during the entire time I was away. Imagine my surprise when I got home, stepped on my bathroom scale, and discovered I'd actually lost three more pounds. It was great motivation to get right back on track once things settled down and got back to normal.

Life happens. *Ten Years Thinner* allows your body to absorb the occasional curve ball without sacrificing everything you've achieved."

— *Jillian, 38*

"Between a work situation and a family illness, there was a month when I wasn't exercising and three weeks when I had very little control over the food I was eating. I stopped looking at myself in the mirror because I didn't want to watch the toll that inactivity was taking on my body. But at the end of the crisis period, I was shocked to find I hadn't gained a pound.

It's obvious to me that the *Ten Years Thinner* program hasn't just increased my metabolism, it's changed how my body processes food. There is a built-in margin of forgiveness so that if you fall off the wagon, you won't start to backslide right away. This program fits with a real life. It's great to know that your efforts won't go to waste the minute you miss a workout!"

— *Matt, 38*

A LIFETIME OF HEALTHY EATING

By now, you know the difference between healthy and unhealthy foods, and you know how and why adequate amounts of healthy macro- and micronutrients are absolutely essential to a firm, youthful physique, high energy levels, and accelerated fat burning. You are ready to learn healthy strategies for dining out, tips for guilt-free indulging during the holiday season, and basic guidelines for alcohol consumption. And it's time to add some treats—like a weekly cheat meal. You read right. From this point forward, you are encouraged to indulge in one cheat meal per week during which you should allow yourself to eat *as much as* you want, of *anything* you want. The only rule is that you limit the duration of this food free-for-all to a maximum of 90 minutes.

Dining Out

Since you shouldn't cheat more than once a week, if you eat out more often than that, you may need to learn some strategies for restaurant dining. It's surprisingly easy to apply the healthy eating guidelines you've learned over the past weeks to restaurant situations:

1. Ask your server not to bring any complimentary bread, rolls, chips, or fried noodles prior to your meal. If they're not there in the first place, you won't be tempted to eat them while you're waiting for your order.

2. Avoid sandwiches, pasta dishes, and fried items in favor of grilled and baked foods.

3. Be sure the meal includes at least a fist's worth of protein. If you're ordering a salad as your entree, this usually means adding a side of grilled chicken breast or shrimp.

4. Whenever possible, request that sauces and creamy dressings be served separately so you can control how much you're using. Limit these items to two tablespoons per meal.

5. Be sure the meal includes one to two fists worth of fruits, vegetables, and/or legumes. The easiest way to do this is usually to ask your server if you can substitute a side salad, fruit salad, or extra vegetables for any

potatoes, chips, fries, rice, bread, pasta, and/or corn that normally come with your entree.

6. Limit alcohol consumption to one drink.

The Holidays

Healthy eating during the holiday season can be a challenge. On the other hand, now that you've gone six weeks with minimal high glycemic foods, you should no longer experience significant cravings. Breads, potatoes, and bread stuffings will not hold the same irresistible allure of yore. Likewise, the cookies, pies, pastries, and other sugary delicacies will no longer seem as tempting as they did last year. Nevertheless, I recommend that both Thanksgiving and Christmas dinner be counted as cheat meals so you are free to indulge. The following list of simple suggestions can help make the holidays more navigable:

1. When the bird hits the table, choose light meat over dark meat.

2. Substitute yams for potatoes.

3. Remember the two tablespoons rule. Avoid the temptation to smother all your food with copious amounts of gravy.

4. Don't starve yourself before the big dinner. The longer you go without eating, the more sluggish your metabolism, and the more likely you are to overeat at your next meal.

5. If you chew slowly and savor your food, you will feel fuller sooner and eat less.

A Word on Alcohol

Where body composition is concerned, I've always maintained that alcohol is the enemy of a firm physique. Alcohol contains 7 calories per gram, nearly twice that found in the equivalent amount of carbohydrate or protein, and is completely without nutritional value. Regular alcohol consumption increases fat retention (especially belly fat), decreases fat burning, diminishes muscle growth and repair, impairs liver function, and decreases cognitive abilities. In addition, although alcohol itself is not believed to be carcinogenic, one of its primary metabolites, a chemical known as *acetaldehyde*, reacts with DNA to promote malignancies.

While many epidemiological studies suggest that moderate alcohol consumption may actually decrease one's risk of death from heart disease, the apparent benefits are offset at higher drinking levels by an increased risk of death from heart disease. For optimal health and a firm physique, alcohol consumption should be limited to a maximum of one drink per day for women, and two for men. If you know ahead of time that you are going to drink to excess, have your booze binge on the same night as your cheat meal.

A LIFETIME OF PHYSICAL ACTIVITY

According to statistics, half of those individuals who begin a new program of regular exercise will abandon it within the first 12 months. Why are the numbers so dismal? Well, for starters, as I alluded to in Chapter 7, most exercise programs fail to provide the promised results. At this juncture, you have firsthand knowledge that the *Ten Years Thinner* exercise routines produce rapid, tangible improvements in body composition. In fact, this may be all the motivation you need to stay active!

Rest assured, the Phase 2 workout will continue to produce improvements in body composition for many weeks to come. Once you reach your ideal weight, I recommend doing the Phase 2 workout at least four times per week to maintain your firm physique. I also strongly encourage you to expand your exercise repertoire by exploring new forms of physical activity. Just remember that the key to achieving and maintaining optimal body composition resides in:

1. toning the muscles throughout your entire body with full-body resistance training; *and*

2. repeatedly elevating your heart rate into the out-of-breath anaerobic zone.

You can accomplish both objectives simultaneously with the *Ten Years Thinner* exercise routines. Alternatively, if you have the time and inclination, you might consider spicing up your workouts by addressing each goal separately with different types of training. For example, you could combine a weight-lifting routine two to three days a week with an outdoor activity two to three days a week. Don't forget, if your activity calls for sustained, low-intensity levels of exertion (like running, cycling, or swimming), you won't reap the benefits of EPOC and accelerated fat burning unless your training sessions are punctuated by brief sprints that periodically drive your heart rate into the out-of-breath anaerobic zone. Many sports, such as hockey, mountain biking, soccer, tennis, and skiing, tend to do this automatically.

Maintaining Motivation

Many experts contend that most people's inability to commit to a long-term exercise program boils down to a lack of long-term motivation. Unfortunately, a lack of motivation is not a simple issue to address. While every person shares certain elements of the human genome, we are each a unique expression of DNA, with our very own innate talents and frailties. Our aptitudes and aversions are shaped by our life experiences, creating an infinite array of impressions, memories, and perceptions. As a result, each of us develops a natural "style" for negotiating through life. There are dozens of ways to stimulate fat loss, promote cardiovascular health, encourage flexibility, and build muscle. Perhaps the key to maintaining an active lifestyle lies in identifying those activities that compliment your unique motivational style.

Having worked with dozens of private fitness clients over the years, I have arrived at the conclusion that, when it comes to exercise, there are three fundamental motivational styles. Although everyone possesses elements of each archetype, most people identify most strongly with one particular style. By recognizing which characteristics approximate your tendencies, you can better design your exercise program for long-term success.

The Hedonist.   The hedonist only likes to do things she considers to be fun. These individuals have an overwhelming tendency to get sidetracked from the task at hand if something more enjoyable presents itself.

Exercise Strategies for Long-Term Success: Designing a workout program should come as second nature for you. Simply listen to your inner child and approach your workouts as if you were going to summer camp. Do things you love! With your oscillating attention span and easy distractibility, engaging in a myriad of activities is a great way to help you maintain enthusiasm for exercise. If you choose to join a health club, pick one with numerous ancillary benefits like exercise classes, swimming, and racket sports.

Specific Recommendations: To prevent monotony, mix your training up with at least one outdoor activity. For example, you might take up rock climbing, learn to skate, or dust off your mountain bike. If you loved to play sports as a kid, join a team. If you look forward to your annual trip to Aspen with giddy excitement, consider making a trek to your local ski hill a weekly event. Remember, the whole key for you is to keep having fun!

The Extrovert.   The extroverted exerciser is a social exerciser who takes pleasure in camaraderie. She thrives on positive feedback and praise for her efforts.

Exercise Strategies for Long-Term Success: Once you feel accepted and approved of, you tend to push yourself to excel. If you choose to join a health club, be sure that it offers group classes and activities like spinning, aerobics, and kickboxing. Don't be afraid to train during peak times; the enjoyment you receive from being part of a large gathering will likely outweigh the inconvenience of having to wait a couple of extra minutes for a piece of equipment. Because you respond especially keenly to praise, coaches, personal trainers, and workout partners can be a powerful source of continuing motivation.

Suggestions for Specific Sports/Activities: Your social aptitude make you especially well suited for team sports, martial arts, fitness/figure, and dance, all of which permit you the opportunity to showcase your skills as you advance in proficiency. If you are more cause-minded than competitive, there are a growing number of charitable foundations that organize training camps and athletic events for the purpose of fund-raising.

The Introvert.   The introverted exerciser sets internal standards, craves challenge and betterment, and derives fulfillment from efforts that support her convictions.

Exercise Strategies for Long-Term Success: The firm belief in the importance of a healthy body may be all that you require to exercise regularly. Although you relish progress, your benchmarks for success are less concrete and more internalized. Goal setting is a powerful motivational technique that compliments your need for perceived advancement. To permit a focused approach to training, short-term goals should be a clearly defined, realistic slice of your long-term objectives; keep a training journal to track your progress. Test the waters carefully before committing to a health club. Be sure that there aren't too many people for your comfort level during the times you plan to train. Donning headphones and listening to your favorite music not only makes your workout more enjoyable, it will discourage unsolicited conversation with other gym members.

Suggestions for Specific Sports/Activities: Although you strive for excellence, you compete primarily with yourself and do not rely heavily on external feedback for motivation. You may find that you prefer solitary sports and activities that take you away from the daily grind and allow you to spend some time lost in thought. Cycling, mountain biking, and cross-country skiing fit the bill.

For more information on exercise alternatives, including advanced movement and tips for adapting the *Ten Years Thinner* exercise routines so you can train around an injury, please visit the *Ten Years Thinner* Web site at www.tenyearsthinner.com.

The Tools

PHASE I:
Diet and Exercise Guidelines for Weeks 1–3

WEEKS 1&2 DIETARY GUIDELINES

General

1. Eat three meals per day. Each meal must include *at least* one serving of lean protein plus *at least* one serving of fruit and/or vegetables.
2. You may season your food with unlimited amounts of any of the unrestricted condiment ingredients listed below.
3. Eat a midmorning and a midafternoon snack. If you finish eating your last meal more than three hours prior to bedtime, you should also eat a pre-bedtime snack.
4. Eat up to 1/2 cup of snack mix plus a piece of fresh fruit at snack times. Create your snack mix according to your own personal preferences. Your snack mix may consist of only a single item, like cashews, or any combination of the nuts and seeds listed below.
5. Drink 10–12 ounces of fluid with each of your meals and snacks.
6. You may also have up to three cups of black coffee or black tea each day. However, these beverages do not count toward the 60+ ounces (about two liters) of fluid you should be drinking each day.
7. All meal ingredients, snack ingredients, and beverage options should be chosen from the food lists provided below.
8. All cooking must be done using cold-pressed, extra-virgin olive oil.

9. Supplement with:

- one high-potency multivitamin every day
- coldwater fish oil or gel-caps, 2–3 grams, twice/day
- calcium 350–500 mg, twice/day
- magnesium 200–400 mg, twice/day

WEEKS 1 & 2 FOOD AND BEVERAGE LISTS

Meal Ingredients

Lean Protein Options (one serving = one fist).   *Include a minimum of one serving of lean protein with each of your three meals.*

Eggs
   free range eggs (3 medium-to-large eggs)
   regular eggs (4 whites plus 2 yolks)
   Egg Beaters

Poultry
   chicken breast (skinless)
   ground chicken or turkey (breast meat only)
   ground chicken or turkey (regular) (browned and drained of fat)
   ostrich
   turkey breast

Meat
   buffalo
   game (moose, elk, venison, etc.)
   lean ground sirloin (browned and drained of fat)
   pork loin trimmed of fat
   sirloin beef tip trimmed of fat

Seafood
   abalone
   bass
   bluefish

carp
catfish
clams
cod
crab
flounder
grouper
haddock
halibut
lobster
octopus
perch
pike
pollock
monkfish
mussels
red snapper
salmon
shark
shrimp
sole
squid
swordfish
trout
tuna
white fish

Fruits and Vegetables. *Include a minimum of one serving of either fruit or vegetables with each of your three meals.*

Fruits (one serving = one fist)
apple
apricot
banana
blackberries
blueberries
boysenberries
cantaloupe

cherries
cranberries
currants
grapefruit
grapes
kiwi
mango
melon (honeydew)
nectarine
orange
papaya
passion fruit
peach
pear
pineapple
plum
raspberries
strawberries
tangerine
watermelon

Vegetables (one serving = two fists unless otherwise specified)

avocado (one serving = 1/2 avocado)
alfalfa sprouts
artichokes
asparagus
bamboo shoots
beets
broccoli
Brussels sprouts
cabbage
carrots
cauliflower
celery
collard greens
cucumber
dandelion greens
eggplant

endive
kale
lettuce
mushrooms
okra
onion
parsnips
peppers
rutabaga
spinach
squash
tomatoes
yams (one serving = 1/2 fist)
zucchini

Condiments.   *You may season your food with unlimited amounts of the following items:*
fresh or dried spices
garlic
horseradish
hot sauce
lemon juice
mustard
olive oil
onion
pepper
pickles
salsa
salt
sesame oil/sesame seeds
vinegar/vinaigrette

Snack Ingredients

Eat up to 1/2 cup of snack mix and a piece of fresh fruit at snack times.

Fruit (one serving = one fist; see list above)
Snack Mix (one serving = 1/2 cup or two small handfuls)
almonds

brazil nuts
cashews
filberts
macadamia nuts
pecans
pistachio nuts
pumpkin seeds
sunflower seeds
hazelnuts
walnuts

Beverage Options

Drink at least 60 ounces (about two liters) of fluids every day. Choose your beverages from the following list:

water
water with lemon, lime, or fresh berry juice
sparkling water
sparkling water with lemon, lime, or fresh berry juice
flavored (unsweetened) sparkling water
iced green tea (3–4 bags per 2 liters is recommended for best taste)
iced herbal tea (3–4 bags per 2 liters is recommended for best taste)

WEEK 3 DIETARY GUIDELINES

** = New Guidelines

General

1. Eat three meals per day. Each meal must include *at least* one serving of lean protein plus *at least* one serving of fruit and/or vegetables.
2. **At the beginning of week 3, low-fat processed meats such as cold cuts and sausages, etc., may be used as protein food options. In order to qualify as low-fat, the total fat content should not exceed about 35 percent of total calories. In other words, there should be at least 4 grams of protein for every gram of fat.
3. **In addition to the fruits and vegetables listed above, legumes (beans, bean sprouts, peas, soybeans, and peanuts) are permitted starting at the beginning of week 3. Legumes may be consumed either as an alternative

to, or in addition to, the fruits and vegetables already listed. Likewise, soybeans and peanuts may now be included as snack mix ingredients.

4. You may season your food with unlimited amounts of any of the condiment ingredients listed below.

5. Eat a midmorning and a midafternoon snack. If you finish eating your last meal more than three hours prior to bedtime, you should also eat a pre-bedtime snack.

6. Eat up to 1/2 cup of snack mix plus a piece of fresh fruit at snack times. Create your snack mix according to your own personal preferences. Your snack mix may consist of only a single item, like cashews, or any combination of the nuts, seeds, and **legumes listed below.

7. Drink 10–12 ounces of fluid with each of your meals and snacks.

8. You may also have up to three cups of black coffee or black tea each day. However, these beverages do not count toward the 60+ ounces (about two liters) of fluid you should be drinking each day.

9. All meal ingredients, snack ingredients, and beverage options should be chosen from the food lists provided below.

10. All cooking must be done using cold-pressed, extra-virgin olive oil.

11. Supplement with:

- one high-potency multivitamin every day
- coldwater fish oil or gel-caps, 2–3 grams, twice/day
- calcium 350–500 mg, twice/day
- magnesium 200–400 mg, twice/day

WEEK 3 FOOD AND BEVERAGE LISTS

** = New Items

Meal Ingredients

Lean Protein Options (one serving = one fist). *Include a minimum of one serving of lean protein with each of your three meals.*

Eggs
free range eggs (3 medium-to-large eggs)
regular eggs (4 whites plus 2 yolks)
Egg Beaters

Poultry
chicken (skinless)
ground chicken or turkey (breast meat only)
ground chicken or turkey (regular) (browned & drained of fat)
ostrich
turkey (skinless)

Meat
buffalo
game (moose, elk, venison, etc.)
lean ground sirloin (browned and drained of fat)
pork loin trimmed of fat
sirloin beef tip trimmed of fat

Seafood
abalone
bass
bluefish
carp
catfish
clams
cod
crab
flounder
grouper
haddock
halibut
lobster
octopus
perch
pike
pollock
monkfish
mussels
red snapper
salmon

shark
shrimp
sole
squid
swordfish
trout
tuna
white fish

Miscellaneous
low-fat processed meats (at least 4 grams of protein per gram of fat)

Fruits, Vegetables, and Legumes.   Include a minimum of one serving of fruit, vegetables, and/or legumes with each of your three meals.

Fruits (one serving = one fist)
apple
apricot
banana
blackberries
blueberries
boysenberries
cantaloupe
cherries
cranberries
currants
grapefruit
grapes
kiwi
mango
melon (honeydew)
nectarine
orange
papaya
passion fruit
peach

pear
pineapple
plum
raspberries
strawberries
tangerine
watermelon

Vegetables (one serving = two fists unless otherwise specified)
avocado (one serving = 1/2 avocado)
alfalfa sprouts
artichokes
asparagus
bamboo shoots
beets
broccoli
Brussels sprouts
cabbage
carrots
cauliflower
celery
collard greens
cucumber
dandelion greens
eggplant
endive
kale
lettuce
mushrooms
okra
onion
parsnips
peppers
rutabaga
spinach
squash
tomatoes

yams (one serving = 1/2 fist)
zucchini

Legumes (one serving = one fist)
  **bean sprouts
  **black beans
  **brown beans
  **fava beans
  **garbanzo beans
  **green beans
  **kidney beans
  **lentils
  **lentil sprouts
  **lima beans
  **navy beans
  **peas/pea pods
  **pinto beans
  **red beans
  **refried beans (fat free)
  **soybeans
  **string beans

Condiments.   *You may season your food with unlimited amounts of the following items.*
  fresh or dried spices
  garlic
  horseradish
  hot sauce
  lemon juice
  mustard
  olive oil
  onion
  pepper
  pickles
  salsa
  salt
  sesame oil/sesame seeds
  vinegar/vinaigrette

Snack Ingredients

Eat up to 1/2 cup of snack mix and a piece of fresh fruit at snack times.

Fruit (one serving = one fist; see list above)
Snack Mix (one serving = 1/2 cup or two small handfuls)
almonds
brazil nuts
cashews
filberts
macadamia nuts
**peanuts
pecans
pistachio nuts
pumpkin seeds
**soybeans
sunflower seeds
hazelnuts
walnuts

Beverage Options

Drink at least 60 ounces (about two liters) of fluids every day. Choose your beverages from the following list:
water
water with lemon, lime, or fresh berry juice
sparkling water
sparkling water with lemon, lime, or fresh berry juice
flavored (unsweetened) sparkling water
iced green tea (3–4 bags per 2 liters recommended for best taste)
iced herbal tea (3–4 bags per 2 liters recommended for best taste)

---♦♦♦---

WEEK 1 EXERCISE ROUTINE

(AMAP = As Many As Possible)

1. step-ups (15x one leg then 15x the opposite leg)
2. novice or regular push-ups (AMAP up to 20x)
3. lunge-curls (AMAP up to 30x alternating legs)
4. squeeze-crunches (AMAP up to 20x)
5. squat-presses (AMAP up to 20x)
6. rows (AMAP up to 20x)
7. squat-raises (AMAP up to 20x)
8. squeeze-side-crunches (AMAP up to 10x/side)
9. novice or regular sissy-squats (AMAP up to 20x)
10. novice, regular, or advanced bench-dips (AMAP up to 20x)
11. calf-raises (AMAP up to 20x)
12. squeeze-crunches (AMAP up to 20x)

5-MINUTE STRETCHING ROUTINE

1. frog-legs (adductor stretch)
2. pie-bows (hamstring stretch)
3. tush-twists (glute stretch)
4. pelicans (quadriceps stretch)
5. rag-dolls (spine stretch)
6. strippers (biceps/chest stretch)
7. towel-tugs (triceps/shoulder stretch)

Photocopy and post this page for easy reference during your workouts.

WEEKS 2 & 3 EXERCISE ROUTINE

(AMAP = As Many As Possible)

1. step-ups (20x one leg then 20x the opposite leg)
2. novice or regular push-ups (AMAP up to 30x)
3. lunge-curls (AMAP up to 40x alternating legs)
4. squeeze-crunches (AMAP up to 30x)
5. squat-presses (AMAP up to 30x)
6. rows (AMAP up to 30x)
7. squat-raises (AMAP up to 30x)
8. squeeze-side-crunches (AMAP up to 15x/side)
9. novice or regular sissy-squats (AMAP up to 30x)
10. novice, regular, or advanced bench-dips (AMAP up to 30x)
11. calf-raises (AMAP up to 30x)
12. squeeze-crunches (AMAP up to 30x)

5-MINUTE STRETCHING ROUTINE

1. frog-legs (adductor stretch)
2. pie-bows (hamstring stretch)
3. tush-twists (glute stretch)
4. pelicans (quadriceps stretch)
5. rag-dolls (spine stretch)
6. strippers (biceps/chest stretch)
7. towel-tugs (triceps/shoulder stretch)

Photocopy and post this page for easy reference during your workouts.

PHASE II:
Diet and Exercise
Guidelines for Weeks 4–6

WEEK 4 DIETARY GUIDELINES

** = New Guidelines

General

1. Eat three meals per day. Each meal must include *at least* one serving of lean protein plus *at least* one serving of fruit, vegetables, and/or legumes.
2. **At the beginning of week four, you may also have up to 100 calories worth of dairy or soy-based foods with each meal. Unless these new food items actually appear on the protein list, they cannot be substituted for a serving of lean protein.**
3. You may season your food with unlimited amounts of any of the unrestricted condiments, **or a total of up to two tablespoons of the restricted condiments listed below.**
4. Eat a midmorning and a midafternoon snack. If you finish eating your last meal more than three hours prior to bedtime, you should also eat a pre-bedtime snack.
5. Eat up to 1/2 cup of snack mix and/or a piece of fresh fruit **and/or 3/4 cup of plain yogurt** at snack times. Create your snack mix according to your own personal preferences. Your snack mix may consist of only a single item, like cashews, or any combination of the nuts, seeds, and legumes listed below.
6. Drink 10–12 ounces of fluid with each of your meals and snacks.

7. All protein foods, fruits and vegetables, snacks, condiments, and beverage items should be chosen from the food lists provided below.
8. All cooking must be done using cold-pressed, extra-virgin olive oil.

Supplement with:

- one high-potency multivitamin every day
- ultra-purified coldwater fish oil or gel-caps, 2–3 grams, twice/day

**If you have one serving or less of dairy (or calcium-fortified food)/day:

- **take 300–500 mg of calcium, twice/day, plus**
- **200–400 mg of magnesium, twice/day**

**If you have two or more servings of dairy (or calcium-fortified food)/day:

- **take 300–350 mg of calcium, once/day, plus**
- **200–400 mg of magnesium, twice/day**

WEEK 4 FOOD AND BEVERAGE LISTS

Meal Ingredients

Lean Protein Options (one serving = one fist).   *Include a minimum of one serving of lean protein with each of your three meals.*

** = New Items

Dairy
  **fat-free or low-fat cottage cheese
  **fat-free or low-fat ricotta cheese

Eggs
  free range eggs (3 medium-to-large eggs)
  regular eggs (4 whites plus 2 yolks)
  Egg Beaters

**Protein Powder (20–25 grams or about
1 heaping scoop for most brands)**
　**egg protein (any flavor)
　**whey protein (any flavor)

Poultry
　chicken (skinless)
　ground chicken or turkey (breast meat only)
　ground chicken or turkey (regular) (browned & drained of fat)
　ostrich
　turkey (skinless)

Meat
　buffalo
　game (moose, elk, venison, etc.)
　lean ground sirloin (browned and drained of fat)
　pork loin trimmed of fat
　sirloin beef tip trimmed of fat

Seafood
　abalone
　bass
　bluefish
　carp
　catfish
　clams
　cod
　crab
　flounder
　grouper
　haddock
　halibut
　lobster
　octopus
　perch
　pike
　pollock

monkfish
mussels
red snapper
salmon
shark
shrimp
sole
squid
swordfish
trout
tuna
white fish

Miscellaneous
low-fat processed meats (at least 4 grams of protein per gram of fat)

Fruits, Vegetables, and Legumes. Include a minimum of one serving of fruit, vegetables, and/or legumes with each of your three meals.

Fruits (one serving = one fist)
apple
apricot
banana
blackberries
blueberries
boysenberries
cantaloupe
cherries
cranberries
currants
grapefruit
grapes
kiwi
mango
melon (honeydew)
nectarine
orange

papaya
passion fruit
peach
pear
pineapple
plum
raspberries
strawberries
tangerine
watermelon

Vegetables (one serving = two fists unless otherwise specified)

avocado (one serving = 1/2 avocado)
alfalfa sprouts
artichokes
asparagus
bamboo shoots
beets
broccoli
Brussels sprouts
cabbage
carrots
cauliflower
celery
collard greens
cucumber
dandelion greens
eggplant
endive
kale
lettuce
mushrooms
okra
onion
parsnips
peppers
rutabaga

spinach
squash
tomatoes
yams (one serving = 1/2 fist)
zucchini

Legumes (one serving = one fist)
bean sprouts
black beans
brown beans
fava beans
garbanzo beans
green beans
kidney beans
lentils
lentil sprouts
lima beans
navy beans
peas/pea pods
pinto beans
red beans
refried beans (fat free)
soybeans
string beans

Dairy and Soy-Based Foods.   *You may also have up to 100 calories worth of dairy or soy-based foods with each of your three meals.*
**skim or 1% milk
**low-fat cheeses
**low-fat sour cream
**low-fat plain yogurt
**tofu
**soy-based meat and dairy substitutes

Unrestricted Condiments.   *You may season your food with unlimited amounts of the following items.*
fresh or dried spices
garlic

horseradish
hot sauce
lemon juice
mustard
olive oil
onion
pepper
pickles
salsa
salt
sesame oil/sesame seeds
vinegar/vinaigrette

Restricted Condiments. *Unless otherwise specified, you may season your food with up to a total of two, level tablespoons (per meal) of any of the following items.*

bacon bits
barbecue sauce
butter (up to one level tablespoon)
cocoa
creamy salad dressing
gravy
marinade
mayo
ground nuts
nut butter (up to one level tablespoon)
peanut butter (up to one level tablespoon)
sauce (including wine sauce, cheese sauce, etc.)
sugar, brown sugar, and honey (small amounts for cooking)
tartar sauce
tomato sauce (up to 1/2 cup)

Snack Ingredients

Eat up to 1/2 cup of snack mix and/or a piece of fresh fruit and/or 3/4 cup of plain yogurt at snack times.

**Plain Yogurt (one serving = 3/4 cup)
Fruit (one serving = one fist; see list above)
Snack Mix (one serving = 1/2 cup or two small handfuls)

almonds
brazil nuts
cashews
filberts
macadamia nuts
peanuts
pecans
pistachio nuts
pumpkin seeds
soybeans
sunflower seeds
hazelnuts
walnuts

Beverage Options

Drink at least 60 ounces (about two liters) of fluids every day. Choose your beverages from the following list:

water
water with lemon, lime, or fresh berry juice
sparkling water
sparkling water with lemon, lime, or fresh berry juice
flavored (unsweetened) sparkling water
iced green tea (3–4 bags per 2 liters recommended for best taste)
iced herbal tea (3–4 bags per 2 liters recommended for best taste)
**unsweetened fruit juice (limit to a TOTAL of 8 oz. [1 cup/day])

WEEKS 5 & 6 DIETARY GUIDELINES

** = New Guidelines

General

1. Eat three meals per day. Each meal must include *at least* one serving of lean protein plus *at least* one serving of fruit, vegetables, and/or legumes.

2. You may also have up to 100 calories worth of dairy or soy-based foods with each meal. Unless these food items actually appear on the protein list, they cannot be substituted for a serving of lean protein.

3. **At the beginning of week 5, you may also have up to 100 calories worth of grain based or high glycemic foods with each meal. These new food items cannot be substituted for the mandatory servings of fruit, vegetables, and/or legumes.**

4. You may season your food with unlimited amounts of any of the unrestricted condiments, or a total of up to two tablespoons of the restricted condiments listed below.

5. Eat a midmorning and a midafternoon snack. If you finish eating your last meal more than three hours prior to bedtime, you should also eat a pre-bedtime snack.

6. Eat up to 1/2 cup of snack mix and/or a piece of fresh fruit and/or 3/4 cup of plain yogurt at snack times. Create your snack mix according to your own personal preferences. Your snack mix may consist of only a single item, like cashews, or any combination of the nuts, seeds, and legumes listed below, **plus up to two ounces of chocolate or dried fruit.**

7. Drink 10–12 ounces of fluid with each of your meals and snacks.

8. All protein foods, fruits and vegetables, snacks, condiments, and beverage items should be chosen from the food lists provided below.

9. All cooking must be done using cold-pressed, extra-virgin olive oil.

10. Supplement with:
    - one high-potency multivitamin every day
    - ultra-purified coldwater fish oil or gel-caps, 2–3 grams, twice/day

If you have one serving or less of dairy (or calcium-fortified food)/day:

- take 300–500 mg of calcium, twice/day, plus
- 200–400 mg of magnesium, twice/day

If you have two or more servings of dairy (or calcium-fortified food)/day:

- take 300–350 mg of calcium, once/day, plus
- 200–400 mg of magnesium, twice/day

WEEKS 5 & 6 FOOD
AND BEVERAGE LISTS

Meal Ingredients

Lean Protein Options (one serving = one fist).   *Include a minimum of one serving of lean protein with each of your three meals.*

** = New Items

Dairy
fat-free or low-fat cottage cheese
fat-free or low-fat ricotta cheese

Eggs
free range eggs (3 medium-to-large eggs)
regular eggs (4 whites plus 2 yolks)
Egg Beaters

Protein Powder (20–25 grams or about 1 heaping scoop for most brands)
egg protein (any flavor)
whey protein (any flavor)

Poultry
chicken (skinless)
ground chicken or turkey (breast meat only)
ground chicken or turkey (regular) (browned & drained of fat)
ostrich
turkey (skinless)

Meat
buffalo
game (moose, elk, venison, etc.)
lean ground sirloin (browned and drained of fat)
pork loin trimmed of fat
sirloin beef tip trimmed of fat

Seafood
> abalone
> bass
> bluefish
> carp
> catfish
> clams
> cod
> crab
> flounder
> grouper
> haddock
> halibut
> lobster
> octopus
> perch
> pike
> pollock
> monkfish
> mussels
> red snapper
> salmon
> shark
> shrimp
> sole
> squid
> swordfish
> trout
> tuna
> white fish

Miscellaneous
> low-fat processed meats (at least 4 grams of protein per gram of fat)

Fruits, Vegetables, and Legumes. *Include a minimum of one serving of fruit, vegetables, and/or legumes with each of your three meals.*

Fruits (one serving = one fist)
apple
apricot
banana
blackberries
blueberries
boysenberries
cantaloupe
cherries
cranberries
currants
grapefruit
grapes
kiwi
mango
melon (honeydew)
nectarine
orange
papaya
passion fruit
peach
pear
pineapple
plum
raspberries
strawberries
tangerine
watermelon

Vegetables (one serving = two fists unless otherwise specified)
avocado (one serving = 1/2 avocado)
alfalfa sprouts
artichokes
asparagus
bamboo shoots
beets
broccoli

Brussels sprouts
cabbage
carrots
cauliflower
celery
collard greens
cucumber
dandelion greens
eggplant
endive
kale
lettuce
mushrooms
okra
onion
parsnips
peppers
rutabaga
spinach
squash
tomatoes
yams (one serving = 1/2 fist)
zucchini

Legumes (one serving = one fist)
bean sprouts
black beans
brown beans
fava beans
garbanzo beans
green beans
kidney beans
lentils
lentil sprouts
lima beans
navy beans
peas/pea pods

pinto beans
red beans
refried beans (fat free)
soybeans
string beans

Dairy and Soy-Based Foods. *You may have up to 100 calories worth of dairy or soy-based foods with each of your three meals.*

skim or 1% milk
low-fat cheeses
low-fat sour cream
low-fat plain yogurt
tofu
soy-based meat and dairy substitutes

Grain-Based and High Glycemic Foods. *You may also have up to 100 calories worth of grain-based or HGI foods with each of your three meals. Reference servings are listed below.*

**whole wheat or whole grain bagel	1/2
**whole wheat or whole grain bread	1 slice
**whole grain cereal	3/4 cup
**corn	1 ear
**oatmeal	1 cup (uncooked)
**whole wheat or rice pasta	1 cup (cooked)
**potato	1 cup
**rice	3/4 cup (cooked)
**whole wheat wrap	1 medium

Unrestricted Condiments. *You may season your food with unlimited amounts of the following items.*

fresh or dried spices
garlic
horseradish
hot sauce
lemon juice
mustard
olive oil

onion
pepper
pickles
salsa
salt
sesame oil/sesame seeds
**soy sauce
vinegar/vinaigrette

Restricted Condiments. Unless otherwise specified, you may season your food with up to a total of two, level tablespoons (per meal) of any of the following items.

bacon bits
barbecue sauce
butter (up to one level tablespoon)
**chocolate syrup
cocoa
creamy salad dressing
**flax seed oil
gravy
honey
**jelly
**jam
marinade
mayo
ground nuts
**maple syrup
nut butter (up to one level tablespoon)
peanut butter (up to one level tablespoon)
sauce (including wine sauce, cheese sauce, etc.)
tartar sauce
tomato sauce (up to 1/2 cup)
**Worcestershire sauce

Snack Ingredients

Eat up to 1/2 cup of snack mix and/or a piece of fresh fruit and/or 3/4 cup of plain yogurt at snack times. Limit chocolate and dried fruit to a total of 2 ounces per snack.

Plain Yogurt (one serving = 3/4 cup)
Fruit (one serving = one fist; see list above)
Snack Mix (one serving = 1/2 cup or two small handfuls)
>   almonds
>   brazil nuts
>   cashews
>   ****coconut shavings (unsweetened)**
>   ****dates**
>   ****dried cranberries**
>   ****dried currants**
>   filberts
>   peanuts
>   pecans
>   pistachio nuts
>   pumpkin seeds
>   ****raisins**
>   ****semi-sweetened chocolate chips**
>   soybeans
>   sunflower seeds
>   hazelnuts
>   walnuts

Beverage Options

Drink at least 60 ounces (about two liters) of fluids every day. Choose your beverages from the following list:
>   water
>   water with lemon, lime, or fresh berry juice
>   sparkling water
>   sparkling water with lemon, lime, or fresh berry juice
>   flavored (unsweetened) sparkling water
>   iced green tea (3–4 bags per 2 liters recommended for best taste)
>   iced herbal tea (3–4 bags per 2 liters recommended for best taste)
>   unsweetened fruit juice **(**limit to a TOTAL of 16 ounces [2 cups/day])**

›››

WEEKS 4–6 EXERCISE ROUTINE

(AMAP = As Many As Possible)

1. step-ups (20x one leg then 20x the opposite leg)
2. rows (30x)
3. lunge-curls (40x alternating legs)
4. squeeze-crunches (30x)
5. horse-curls (20–30x)
6. push-ups (AMAP up to 30x)
7. squat-presses (30x)
8. squeeze-side-crunches (15x/side)
9. squat-raises (30x)
10. rows (30x)
11. wide sissy-squats (30x)
12. squeeze-crunches (30x)
13. standard sissy-squats (30x)
14. bench-dips (AMAP up to 30x)
15. calf-raises (30x)
16. squeeze-side-crunches (30x)

5-MINUTE STRETCHING ROUTINE

1. frog-legs (adductor stretch)
2. pie-bows (hamstring stretch)
3. tush-twists (glute stretch)
4. pelicans (quadriceps stretch)
5. rag-dolls (spine stretch)
6. strippers (biceps/chest stretch)
7. towel-tugs (triceps/shoulder stretch)

Photocopy and post this page for easy reference during your workouts.

♦♦♦

OPTIONAL 30-MINUTE EXERCISE ROUTINE

(AMAP = As Many As Possible)

1. step-ups (20x one leg then 20x the opposite leg)
2. rows (30x)
3. lunge-curls (40x alternating legs)
4. squeeze-crunches (30x)
5. horse curls (20–30x)
6. push-ups (AMAP up to 30x)
7. squat-presses (30x)
8. squeeze-side-crunches (15x/side)
9. squat-raises (30x)
10. rows (30x)
11. wide sissy-squats (30x)
12. squeeze-crunches (30x)
13. reverse lunge-front-raises (30x)
14. push ups or bench push ups (AMAP to 30x)
15. squat thrusts (30x)
16. squeeze-side-crunches (30x)
17. standard sissy-squats (30x)
18. bench-dips (AMAP up to 30x)
19. calf-raises (30x)
20. squeeze-crunches (30x)

5-MINUTE STRETCHING ROUTINE

1. frog-legs (adductor stretch)
2. pie-bows (hamstring stretch)
3. tush-twists (glute stretch)
4. pelicans (quadriceps stretch)
5. rag-dolls (spine stretch)
6. strippers (biceps/chest stretch)
7. towel-tugs (triceps/shoulder stretch)

Photocopy and post this page for easy reference during your workouts.

Self Tracking

COMPLIANCE FORMS

Most program participants found that filling out the compliance forms each day helped keep them honest. Photocopy the form corresponding to the appropriate week and post it where you can see it.

For meals and snacks: Bearing in mind that you shouldn't go more than two and a half hours without eating something, record the times that you have your meals and snacks.

For supplements: Check off each supplement as you take it.

Exercise routine: The compliance forms list the appropriate exercise routine with rest days indicated.

A blank compliance form is included on page 218 if you wish to continue using the log after week 6.

TRACKING YOUR PROGRESS

Program participants also found it very motivating to record the changes in their physiques as the inches melted away. The progress sheet found on page 219 makes this simple to do for the duration of Phases I and II. A blank progress sheet is included on page 220 if you wish to continue tracking your progress after week 6.

WEEK 1

DAY 1	TIME	DAY 2	TIME	DAY 3	TIME	DAY 4	TIME	DAY 5	TIME	DAY 6	TIME	DAY 7	TIME
Meal 1		Meal 1		Meal 1		Meal 1		Meal 1		Meal 1		Meal 1	
Snack 1		Snack 1		Snack 1		Snack 1		Snack 1		Snack 1		Snack 1	
Meal 2		Meal 2		Meal 2		Meal 2		Meal 2		Meal 2		Meal 2	
Snack 2		Snack 2		Snack 2		Snack 2		Snack 2		Snack 2		Snack 2	
Meal 3		Meal 3		Meal 3		Meal 3		Meal 3		Meal 3		Meal 3	
Snack 3 (optional)		Snack 3 (optional)		Snack 3 (optional)		Snack 3 (optional)		Snack 3 (optional)		Snack 3 (optional)		Snack 3 (optional)	
SUPPLEMENTS		SUPPLEMENTS		SUPPLEMENTS		SUPPLEMENTS		SUPPLEMENTS		SUPPLEMENTS		SUPPLEMENTS	
Multi		Multi		Multi		Multi		Multi		Multi		Multi	
Calcium		Calcium		Calcium		Calcium		Calcium		Calcium		Calcium	
Magnesium		Magnesium		Magnesium		Magnesium		Magnesium		Magnesium		Magnesium	
Fish oil		Fish oil		Fish oil		Fish oil		Fish oil		Fish oil		Fish oil	
Week 1 Routine		Week 1 Routine		REST		Week 1 Routine		Week 1 Routine		Week 1 Routine		REST	

WEEK 2
〉〉〉〉〉

DAY 8	TIME	DAY 9	TIME	DAY 10	TIME	DAY 11	TIME	DAY 12	TIME	DAY 13	TIME	DAY 14	TIME
Meal 1		Meal 1		Meal 1		Meal 1		Meal 1		Meal 1		Meal 1	
Snack 1		Snack 1		Snack 1		Snack 1		Snack 1		Snack 1		Snack 1	
Meal 2		Meal 2		Meal 2		Meal 2		Meal 2		Meal 2		Meal 2	
Snack 2		Snack 2		Snack 2		Snack 2		Snack 2		Snack 2		Snack 2	
Meal 3		Meal 3		Meal 3		Meal 3		Meal 3		Meal 3		Meal 3	
Snack 3 (optional)		Snack 3 (optional)		Snack 3 (optional)		Snack 3 (optional)		Snack 3 (optional)		Snack 3 (optional)		Snack 3 (optional)	
SUPPLEMENTS		SUPPLEMENTS		SUPPLEMENTS		SUPPLEMENTS		SUPPLEMENTS		SUPPLEMENTS		SUPPLEMENTS	
Multi		Multi		Multi		Multi		Multi		Multi		Multi	
Calcium		Calcium		Calcium		Calcium		Calcium		Calcium		Calcium	
Magnesium		Magnesium		Magnesium		Magnesium		Magnesium		Magnesium		Magnesium	
Fish oil		Fish oil		Fish oil		Fish oil		Fish oil		Fish oil		Fish oil	
Week 2/3 Routine		Week 2/3 Routine		Week 2/3 Routine		Week 2/3 Routine		REST		Week 2/3 Routine		Week 2/3 Routine	

WEEK 3

DAY 15	TIME	DAY 16	TIME	DAY 17	TIME	DAY 18	TIME	DAY 19	TIME	DAY 20	TIME	DAY 21	TIME
Meal 1		Meal 1		Meal 1		Meal 1		Meal 1		Meal 1		Meal 1	
Snack 1		Snack 1		Snack 1		Snack 1		Snack 1		Snack 1		Snack 1	
Meal 2		Meal 2		Meal 2		Meal 2		Meal 2		Meal 2		Meal 2	
Snack 2		Snack 2		Snack 2		Snack 2		Snack 2		Snack 2		Snack 2	
Meal 3		Meal 3		Meal 3		Meal 3		Meal 3		Meal 3		Meal 3	
Snack 3 (optional)		Snack 3 (optional)		Snack 3 (optional)		Snack 3 (optional)		Snack 3 (optional)		Snack 3 (optional)		Snack 3 (optional)	
SUPPLEMENTS		**SUPPLEMENTS**		**SUPPLEMENTS**		**SUPPLEMENTS**		**SUPPLEMENTS**		**SUPPLEMENTS**		**SUPPLEMENTS**	
Multi		Multi		Multi		Multi		Multi		Multi		Multi	
Calcium		Calcium		Calcium		Calcium		Calcium		Calcium		Calcium	
Magnesium		Magnesium		Magnesium		Magnesium		Magnesium		Magnesium		Magnesium	
Fish oil		Fish oil		Fish oil		Fish oil		Fish oil		Fish oil		Fish oil	
Week 2/3 Routine		Week 2/3 Routine		REST		Week 2/3 Routine		Week 2/3 Routine		Week 2/3 Routine		Week 2/3 Routine	

WEEK 4
ʾʾʾʾʾ

DAY 22	TIME	DAY 23	TIME	DAY 24	TIME	DAY 25	TIME	DAY 26	TIME	DAY 27	TIME	DAY 28	TIME
Meal 1		Meal 1		Meal 1		Meal 1		Meal 1		Meal 1		Meal 1	
Snack 1		Snack 1		Snack 1		Snack 1		Snack 1		Snack 1		Snack 1	
Meal 2		Meal 2		Meal 2		Meal 2		Meal 2		Meal 2		Meal 2	
Snack 2		Snack 2		Snack 2		Snack 2		Snack 2		Snack 2		Snack 2	
Meal 3		Meal 3		Meal 3		Meal 3		Meal 3		Meal 3		Meal 3	
Snack 3 (optional)		Snack 3 (optional)		Snack 3 (optional)		Snack 3 (optional)		Snack 3 (optional)		Snack 3 (optional)		Snack 3 (optional)	
SUPPLEMENTS		**SUPPLEMENTS**		**SUPPLEMENTS**		**SUPPLEMENTS**		**SUPPLEMENTS**		**SUPPLEMENTS**		**SUPPLEMENTS**	
Multi		Multi		Multi		Multi		Multi		Multi		Multi	
Calcium		Calcium		Calcium		Calcium		Calcium		Calcium		Calcium	
Magnesium		Magnesium		Magnesium		Magnesium		Magnesium		Magnesium		Magnesium	
Fish oil		Fish oil		Fish oil		Fish oil		Fish oil		Fish oil		Fish oil	
REST		Phase 2 Routine		Phase 2 Routine		Phase 2 Routine		Phase 2 Routine		**REST**		Phase 2 Routine	

WEEK 5 ‹‹‹‹

DAY 29	TIME	DAY 30	TIME	DAY 31	TIME	DAY 32	TIME	DAY 33	TIME	DAY 34	TIME	DAY 35	TIME
Meal 1		Meal 1		Meal 1		Meal 1		Meal 1		Meal 1		Meal 1	
Snack 1		Snack 1		Snack 1		Snack 1		Snack 1		Snack 1		Snack 1	
Meal 2		Meal 2		Meal 2		Meal 2		Meal 2		Meal 2		Meal 2	
Snack 2		Snack 2		Snack 2		Snack 2		Snack 2		Snack 2		Snack 2	
Meal 3		Meal 3		Meal 3		Meal 3		Meal 3		Meal 3		Meal 3	
Snack 3 (optional)		Snack 3 (optional)		Snack 3 (optional)		Snack 3 (optional)		Snack 3 (optional)		Snack 3 (optional)		Snack 3 (optional)	
SUPPLEMENTS		SUPPLEMENTS		SUPPLEMENTS		SUPPLEMENTS		SUPPLEMENTS		SUPPLEMENTS		SUPPLEMENTS	
Multi		Multi		Multi		Multi		Multi		Multi		Multi	
Calcium		Calcium		Calcium		Calcium		Calcium		Calcium		Calcium	
Magnesium		Magnesium		Magnesium		Magnesium		Magnesium		Magnesium		Magnesium	
Fish oil		Fish oil		Fish oil		Fish oil		Fish oil		Fish oil		Fish oil	
Phase 2 Routine		Phase 2 Routine		Phase 2 Routine		REST		Phase 2 Routine		Phase 2 Routine		Phase 2 Routine	

WEEK 6

DAY 36		DAY 37		DAY 38		DAY 39		DAY 40		DAY 41		DAY 42	
	TIME		TIME		TIME		TIME		TIME		TIME		TIME
Meal 1		Meal 1		Meal 1		Meal 1		Meal 1		Meal 1		Meal 1	
Snack 1		Snack 1		Snack 1		Snack 1		Snack 1		Snack 1		Snack 1	
Meal 2		Meal 2		Meal 2		Meal 2		Meal 2		Meal 2		Meal 2	
Snack 2		Snack 2		Snack 2		Snack 2		Snack 2		Snack 2		Snack 2	
Meal 3		Meal 3		Meal 3		Meal 3		Meal 3		Meal 3		Meal 3	
Snack 3 (optional)		Snack 3 (optional)		Snack 3 (optional)		Snack 3 (optional)		Snack 3 (optional)		Snack 3 (optional)		Snack 3 (optional)	
SUPPLEMENTS		SUPPLEMENTS		SUPPLEMENTS		SUPPLEMENTS		SUPPLEMENTS		SUPPLEMENTS		SUPPLEMENTS	
Multi		Multi		Multi		Multi		Multi		Multi		Multi	
Calcium		Calcium		Calcium		Calcium		Calcium		Calcium		Calcium	
Magnesium		Magnesium		Magnesium		Magnesium		Magnesium		Magnesium		Magnesium	
Fish oil		Fish oil		Fish oil		Fish oil		Fish oil		Fish oil		Fish oil	
Phase 2 Routine		REST		Phase 2 Routine		Phase 2 Routine		Phase 2 Routine		Phase 2 Routine		REST	

WEEK _____

	SUNDAY	TIME	MONDAY	TIME	TUESDAY	TIME	WEDNESDAY	TIME	THURSDAY	TIME	FRIDAY	TIME	SATURDAY	TIME
	Meal 1		Meal 1		Meal 1		Meal 1		Meal 1		Meal 1		Meal 1	
	Snack 1		Snack 1		Snack 1		Snack 1		Snack 1		Snack 1		Snack 1	
	Meal 2		Meal 2		Meal 2		Meal 2		Meal 2		Meal 2		Meal 2	
	Snack 2		Snack 2		Snack 2		Snack 2		Snack 2		Snack 2		Snack 2	
	Meal 3		Meal 3		Meal 3		Meal 3		Meal 3		Meal 3		Meal 3	
	Snack 3 (optional)		Snack 3 (optional)		Snack 3 (optional)		Snack 3 (optional)		Snack 3 (optional)		Snack 3 (optional)		Snack 3 (optional)	
SUPPLEMENTS			SUPPLEMENTS		SUPPLEMENTS		SUPPLEMENTS		SUPPLEMENTS		SUPPLEMENTS		SUPPLEMENTS	
	Multi		Multi		Multi		Multi		Multi		Multi		Multi	
	Calcium		Calcium		Calcium		Calcium		Calcium		Calcium		Calcium	
	Magnesium		Magnesium		Magnesium		Magnesium		Magnesium		Magnesium		Magnesium	
	Fish oil		Fish oil		Fish oil		Fish oil		Fish oil		Fish oil		Fish oil	
Train/Rest			Train/Rest		Train/Rest		Train/Rest		Train/Rest		Train/Rest		Train/Rest	

Appendix C

TRACKING YOUR PROGRESS

For consistency, use the widest part of your body when measuring chest and hips. For waist measurements, use your navel as a landmark. Limit weigh-ins to once a week (or less!) and always weigh yourself first thing in the morning.

DAY 1/Week 1 (Day 1)	Chest: Weight:	Waist:	Hips:
DAY 1/Week 2 (Day 8)	Chest: Weight:	Waist:	Hips:
DAY 1/Week 3 (Day 15)	Chest: Weight:	Waist:	Hips:
DAY 1/Week 4 (Day 22)	Chest: Weight:	Waist:	Hips:
DAY 1/Week 5 (Day 29)	Chest: Weight:	Waist:	Hips:
DAY 1/Week 6 (Day 36)	Chest: Weight:	Waist:	Hips:
DAY 1/Week 7 (Day 43)	Chest: Weight:	Waist:	Hips:

TRACKING YOUR PROGRESS

Date:	Chest: Weight:	Waist:	Hips:
Date:	Chest: Weight:	Waist:	Hips:
Date:	Chest: Weight:	Waist:	Hips:
Date:	Chest: Weight:	Waist:	Hips:
Date:	Chest: Weight:	Waist:	Hips:
Date:	Chest: Weight:	Waist:	Hips:
Date:	Chest: Weight:	Waist:	Hips:
Date:	Chest: Weight:	Waist:	Hips:
Date:	Chest: Weight:	Waist:	Hips:
Date:	Chest: Weight:	Waist:	Hips:

The Ten Years Thinner Recipes

RECIPES FOR WEEKS 1–6

> For more program compliant recipes, please visit the *Ten Years Thinner* Web site at www.tenyearsthinner.com.

Rainbow Salad

Prep time: about 15 minutes

Number of servings as described: approximately 4 full servings of vegetables

Salad Ingredients:

1 pre-washed bag of salad greens

1 pre-washed bag of spinach

5 pre-peeled mini carrots, shredded or grated

1 cup fresh strawberries, thinly sliced

1 cup fresh whole blueberries or whole raspberries

1 red or yellow bell pepper, chopped to bite-size pieces

10 grape or cherry tomatoes, cut in half

1/3 red onion, thinly sliced with rings cut in half

1/2 cucumber, peeled and sliced (English cucumbers do not require peeling)

1 avocado, peeled and cubed

1/2 cup toasted pine nuts or walnuts

In a large bowl, combine and toss salad greens, spinach, berries, carrots, berries, pepper, tomatoes, onion, cucumber, and avocado. Top with toasted pine or walnuts and add salad dressing (see below) to taste.

Dressing Ingredients:

1 part apple cider vinegar

1 part mustard

salt and pepper to taste

Blend until creamy.

Rainbow Salad with Chicken: To turn this salad into 4 full meals, toss with 4 large grilled or broiled skinless, boneless chicken breasts, cubed or sliced into bite-size pieces.

Five-Minute Salad

Prep time: about
5 minutes

Number of servings as
described: 2 full
servings of vegetables

Salad Ingredients:

1 medium tomato, cubed

1 medium avocado, peeled and cubed

1 cucumber, peeled and cubed (English cucumbers do
not require peeling)

1 tablespoon olive oil

juice from 1/2 lemon

ground pepper to taste

dash seasoned salt (optional)

In a medium bowl, combine all ingredients.

Five-Minute Prawn Salad: To turn this salad into 2 full meals, top with 3/4 pound cooked, peeled, and deveined prawns.

♦♦♦♦♦

Painter's Fruit Salad

Prep time: about 10
minutes

Number of servings as
described: about 6
servings of fruit

Salad Ingredients:

1 banana, sliced

2 large Granny Smith apples, peeled, cored, and cubed

1 cup seedless green or red grapes, cut in half

1/2 cantaloupe, gutted and cut into bite-sized pieces

2 kiwis, peeled and cubed

juice of 1/2 lemon

Combine banana, apple, and lemon juice in resealable bag and shake. Empty contents of bag into a medium bowl, add grape halves, cantaloupe, and kiwi. Makes a great dessert, snack, or side with scrambled eggs.

Italian Omelette _____

Prep time: about
5 minutes

Cook time: 5–7
minutes

Number of servings as
described: 1 full meal

Ingredients:
3 eggs
2 tablespoons sun-dried tomatoes in extra-virgin olive oil
1/4 portobello mushroom, thinly sliced
1/2 avocado, peeled and sliced
1/4 cup water
2 tablespoons extra-virgin olive oil (if possible, from jar
of sun-dried tomatoes)
fresh ground pepper

Beat three eggs with 1/4 cup water until slightly frothy. On medium heat in a medium skillet, sauté mushroom and tomatoes in extra-virgin olive oil until tender. Reduce heat, add egg mixture, and cover. Cook until eggs are fluffy but solid. Add avocado, and fold in half. Top with fresh ground pepper to taste.

Tuna Stuffed Tomatoes _____

Prep time: about
5 minutes

Number of servings as
described: 1 full meal

Ingredients:
1 can light tuna in water
2 medium tomatoes, halved and gutted
1 medium celery stalk, chopped
1 tablespoon sesame oil
1/8 teaspoon dill
1/8 teaspoon lemon pepper

Drain tuna. In a small bowl, combine tuna, celery, sesame oil, dill, and pepper to taste. Place one-quarter of mixture into each tomato half.

After Week 4: Add 1/4 cup reduced or nonfat cottage cheese to each cored tomato half before topping with tuna mixture.

Lettuce-Wrap Tacos _____

Prep time: about
10 minutes

Cooking time: about
12 minutes

Number of servings
as described:
approximately
4 full meals

Ingredients:

1½ pounds extra lean ground beef, ground buffalo, or
    ground moose
1 onion, finely chopped
2 tablespoons sliced jalapeño peppers
1 cup sliced black olives
2 medium avocados, peeled and sliced
1 tomato, diced
1 cup fresh or jarred salsa
2 tablespoons taco seasoning
2 tablespoons extra-virgin olive oil
1 head of large-leaf lettuce

Heat 2 tablespoons extra-virgin olive oil in a large skillet over medium heat. Add ground meat, chopped onion, jalapeno peppers, and taco seasoning. Cook until meat is well browned, stirring frequently. Place mixture onto lettuce leaf. Top with salsa, tomato, black olives, and avocado slices. Roll up lettuce leaf and enjoy.

————————————————————————— ❯❯❯❯❯ —————————————————————————

Sole Fillets with Zucchini_____

Prep time: 5–10
minutes

Cooking time: 10–15
minutes depending on
thickness of fillets

Number of servings
as described:
approximately 4
full meals

Ingredients:

4 (6-oz. each) sole fillets
2 medium zucchinis, sliced in 1/2″ rounds
2 cups nonfat, sodium-reduced chicken broth
1 celery stalk, finely chopped
1 red bell pepper, chopped into
    bite-sized pieces
pinch red pepper flakes

In a large skillet or pot, place all ingredients. If necessary, add just enough water that there is sufficient liquid to completely cover the fish. Bring to a boil, then reduce heat, cover, and simmer until fish is no longer opaque and flakes easily.

Roasted Chicken and Yams

Prep time:
5–10 minutes

Cooking time:
60 minutes

Number of servings
as described:
approximately 8
full meals

Ingredients

8–10 skinless boneless chicken breasts

2 large yams, peeled and sliced into 1/2″-thick
    fries or rounds

2 cups nonfat, sodium-reduced chicken broth

1/2 cup extra-virgin olive oil

4 cloves garlic, peeled and minced

1½ tablespoons herbs de provence

Preheat oven to 400 degrees. In a large bowl, combine extra-virgin olive oil, chicken stock, and dry spices. Place yam slices evenly onto the bottom of a 9″ × 12″ casserole dish. Lay chicken breasts flat over yams and pour extra-virgin olive oil/chicken broth mixture over chicken. If necessary, add just enough water so that there is sufficient liquid to completely cover the chicken. Place on middle rack of preheated oven and bake for one hour.

— ✦✦✦✦✦ —

Double Chicken Soup

Prep time: about
10 minutes

Cooking time: about
70 minutes

Number of servings
as described:
approximately 4
full meals

Ingredients:

1½ pounds skinless boneless chicken breast, cubed

3 cloves fresh garlic, minced

2 onions, cut into bite-sized pieces

1 cup celery, chopped into 1/4″ pieces

1/4 cup carrots, chopped into 1/4″ rounds

1 quart (4 cups) non fat, sodium-reduced chicken broth

2 cups water

1/2 teaspoon fresh ground pepper

2 tablespoons extra-virgin olive oil

Heat extra-virgin olive oil in a large pot over medium heat. Add chicken and garlic. Sauté chicken in garlic for five minutes, stirring frequently. Add remaining ingredients and bring to a boil. Reduce to low-medium heat. Cover and simmer for 60 minutes, stirring occasionally.

Quick Fix Chicken Stir Fry

Prep time: about
10 minutes

Cooking time:
10–15 minutes

Number of servings
as described:
approximately 4
full meals

Ingredients

1½ pounds skinless boneless chicken breast, cubed

4 cups fresh or frozen broccoli florets

1 cup fresh or frozen pearl onions

6–8 fresh mushrooms, quartered

1 red bell pepper, cut into bite-sized pieces

1 yellow or orange bell pepper, cut into bite-sized pieces

1 can water chestnuts, drained and sliced

2 tablespoons fresh ginger, minced

4 cloves fresh garlic, minced

4 tablespoons extra-virgin olive oil, divided in 2

2 tablespoons sesame oil, divided in 2

sesame seeds

fresh ground pepper

salt

Heat 2 tablespoons extra-virgin olive oil in a large skillet over medium heat. Add chicken, garlic, and ginger. Cook until chicken is tender and lightly browned on all sides, stirring frequently. Add broccoli, onions, mushrooms, peppers, water chestnuts, and remaining olive and sesame oil. Continue to stir-fry until vegetables reach desired consistency. Top with ground pepper, sesame seeds, and salt to taste.

Eggplant-accini Salad

Prep Time: about
5 minutes

Cooking time:
5–7 minutes

Servings as described:
2–3 servings of
vegetables

Ingredients:

1 eggplant, sliced into 1/4″ rounds

2–3 medium tomatoes, sliced thinly

2 cloves garlic, minced

2 tablespoons fresh chopped basil, divided

extra-virgin olive oil

Balsamic vinegar to taste

Heat about 1/8″ olive oil in a large or medium skillet over low-medium heat. Add garlic, 1 tablespoon fresh basil, and eggplant. Fry eggplant about five minutes per side, until lightly browned. Serve eggplant hot, topped with sliced tomato and garnished with remainder of fresh basil. Drizzle with Balsamic vinegar and olive oil to taste.

Seafood Kabobs

Prep time: about 15 minutes, plus 2 hours to marinate

Cook time: about 10 minutes

Number of servings as described: approximately 4 full meals

Ingredients

3/4 pound raw sea scallops
3/4 pound raw prawns, peeled and deveined
8–10 large fresh mushrooms, cut in half
1 red bell pepper, cut into bite-sized pieces
1 yellow bell pepper, cut into bite-sized pieces
1 green pepper, cut into bite-sized pieces
2 medium onions, cut into bite-sized pieces
2 medium zucchinis, sliced into 1/2″ rounds
3/4 cup extra-virgin olive oil
1 tablespoon Italian Seasoning
2 cloves garlic, peeled and crushed or minced
juice of 1/2 lemon

Combine extra-virgin olive oil, dry spices, garlic, and lemon juice in a resealable bag. Add scallops and prawns, shake, and refrigerate for two hours. After marinating, discard marinade and assemble kabobs evenly using scallops, prawns, mushrooms, peppers, onions, and zucchini. Baste kabobs generously with plain extra-virgin olive oil. Grill or broil until scallops and prawns are opaque.

For Chicken Kabobs, substitute seafood with 1$^1/_2$ pounds skinless, boneless chicken breast cut into 1″ chunks.

———————————————— ❧❧❧❧❧ ————————————————

Yam Frites

Prep Time: about 5 minutes

Cooking time: about 35 minutes

Servings as described: 2–3 servings of vegetables

Ingredients:

1 medium-sized yam, scrubbed and sliced into 1/2″-thick fries
2 egg yolks
1/4 cup extra-virgin olive oil
1/2 teaspoon seasoning salt
1/2 teaspoon cayenne pepper

Preheat oven to 350 degrees. In a small bowl, use whisk to blend egg yolk, extra-virgin olive oil, seasoning salt, and cayenne pepper. Place yam fries in a resealable plastic bag, pour in egg mixture, and shake well. Lay fries onto a cookie sheet that has been lightly greased with extra-virgin olive oil. Bake for 30–40 minutes, or until fries are tender and starting to brown.

Appendix D

RECIPES FOR WEEKS 3–6

....

Chicken Black Bean Salad

Prep time: 10–15 minutes, plus one hour to chill

Cooking time: 5–7 minutes

Number of servings as described: approximately 3 full meals

Ingredients:

1 lb. skinless boneless chicken breast, cubed

2 cups black beans, drained and well rinsed

1 tomato, cubed

1 red bell pepper, chopped into small pieces

1/2 cup green onions, chopped finely

1 avocado, peeled, pitted, and cubed

3 cloves garlic, minced

1/4 teaspoon rubbed basil

1/4 teaspoon ground cumin

1/4 cup fresh chopped cilantro

juice of 1 lemon

4 tablespoons extra-virgin olive oil, divided in two

fresh ground pepper to taste

salt to taste

Heat 2 tablespoons extra-virgin olive oil in a medium skillet over medium heat. Add chicken and garlic. Cook until chicken is tender and lightly browned on all sides, stirring frequently. Transfer chicken to a large bowl and add remaining ingredients. Mix thoroughly and chill in refrigerator for an hour before serving. Salt and pepper to taste.

Salad on Wheels

Prep time: about 10 minutes plus 30 minutes to chill

Number of servings as described: approximately 4 servings of vegetables

Ingredients:

2 cups canned garbanzo beans, drained and rinsed, chilled in refrigerator for at least 1 hour

1 cup frozen green peas, defrosted

1 cucumber, peeled, quartered lengthwise, and cut into 1/4″ slices

1 avocado, peeled and cubed

1/2 cup roasted red peppers, cut into 1/2″ pieces

1 cup black olives, pitted and sliced

In a large salad bowl, combine all ingredients. Add desired amount of dressing (see below). And pepper to taste. Chill for 30 minutes in refrigerator before serving.

Dressing Ingredients:

1/4 cup extra-virgin olive oil

1/4 cup balsamic vinegar

1 tablespoon dry cilantro

1 tablespoon rubbed basil

1 tablespoon cumin

1 teaspoon freshly ground black pepper

2 cloves garlic, minced

1 tablespoon Dijon mustard

Combine dressing ingredients in a shaker bottle and shake well before pouring over salad.

Egg Salad on Wheels: To turn this salad into a full meal, top each serving with two, thinly sliced hard-boiled eggs.

After week 4, top Salad on Wheels with 1/2 cup crumbled feta cheese.

Chili Con Yummy _____

Prep time: about
25 minutes

Cooking time: about
50 minutes

Number of servings
as described:
approximately 6
full meals

Ingredients:

1$\frac{1}{2}$ lbs. skinless, boneless, chicken breast (or lean
     sirloin tip trimmed of visible fat), cubed

3 cups red kidney beans, drained and rinsed

4 cloves garlic, minced

1 cup celery, cut into 1/4″ slices

1$\frac{1}{2}$ cups canned or stewed tomatoes

1/2 cup extra-virgin olive oil

3 tablespoons chili powder

1/2 tablespoon oregano

1/2 tablespoon cumin

1 teaspoon sage

Combine all ingredients in a large pot and bring to a boil. Reduce to low/medium heat. Cover and simmer, stirring frequently for 45 minutes until thick.

Split Pea Soup with Smoked Bratwurst _____

Prep time: 5 minutes

Cooking time: about
45 minutes

Number of servings
as described:
approximately 4
full meals

Ingredients:

1 package (4 links) low-fat bratwurst

2 cups dry green split peas

2 carrots, cut into 1/4″ rounds

1 onion, finely chopped

2 cups nonfat, sodium-reduced chicken broth

5 cups water

1 bay leaf

1$\frac{1}{2}$ teaspoon savory

Quarter bratwurst links lengthwise and cut into 1/2″ pieces. Heat a medium skillet over medium heat and cook bratwurst until lightly browned, stirring frequently. Transfer bratwurst to a large pot. Add all remaining ingredients and bring to a boil. Reduce heat, cover, and simmer for 30–40 minutes, stirring occasionally.

Three-Bean Salad

Prep time: 5 minutes

Number of servings as described: approximately 5 servings of vegetables

Ingredients:

2 cups chickpeas, drained and well rinsed

1 cup kidney beans, drained and well rinsed

1 cup lentils, drained and well rinsed

1 cup broccoli florets

1 red pepper, chopped into small, bite-sized pieces

1 cup salsa

4 tablespoons extra-virgin olive oil

1 tablespoon cumin

Combine all ingredients in a large bowl. Mix well and chill for 30 minutes in the refrigerator before serving.

RECIPES FOR WEEKS 4–6

....

Asparagus Cheese Omelette

Prep time: 5 minutes

Cooking time: 7–10 minutes

Number of servings as described: 1 full meal

Ingredients:
3 eggs
4–6 asparagus spears, tough ends broken off and discarded
1 small tomato, thinly sliced
5 oz. reduced-fat feta cheese
1/4 cup water
2 tablespoons extra-virgin olive oil
fresh ground pepper

Beat three eggs with 1/4 cup water until slightly frothy. On medium heat in a medium skillet, sauté tomato and asparagus in extra-virgin olive oil until asparagus is al dente. Reduce heat, add egg mixture, and top with crumbled cheese. Cook until egg is fluffy but solid. Fold in half and serve topped with fresh ground pepper to taste.

Indian Chicken _____

Prep time: 10–15 minutes

Cooking time: 60 minutes

Number of servings as described: approximately 8 full meals

Ingredients

8–10 skinless chicken hindquarters (thighs and legs)

6 cups chickpeas, mashed

2 cups baby cut carrots

Sauce Ingredients

1½ cups chopped onion

3 cloves garlic, minced

3/4 cup low- or nonfat sour cream

3/4 cup plain nonfat yogurt

5½ oz. tomato paste

1 cup nonfat, sodium reduced chicken broth

1/2 cup extra-virgin olive oil

2 tablespoons curry powder

1/4 teaspoon ground cloves

1 cup frozen peas

Preheat oven to 400 degrees. Lay chicken pieces flat over bottom of 9″ × 12″ casserole dish. Spread mashed chickpeas and baby carrots evenly between and over chicken quarters.

In a large sauce pan, sauté onions and garlic in 2 tablespoons extra-virgin olive oil until onions are clear. Add remaining sauce ingredients and stir over low heat until mixture is well blended. Pour sauce over chicken, baby carrots, and mashed chickpeas. Place on middle rack of preheated oven and bake for one hour.

———————————— ▪▪▪▪▪ ————————————

Turkey Loaf _____

Prep time: about 20 minutes plus 20 minutes to cool

Cooking time: 60 minutes

Number of servings as described: approximately 4 full meals

Ingredients:

1½ pounds ground turkey

2 cups garbanzo beans, mashed

1 cup grated carrot

1 onion, diced

3 cloves garlic, minced

2 tablespoons tomato paste

2 large eggs, lightly beaten

2 tablespoons Worcestershire sauce

1 tablespoon brown sugar

2 tablespoons fresh dill

1/2 teaspoon seasoning salt

3 tablespoons extra-virgin olive oil, divided 2:1

In a small skillet, sauté carrot, onion, and garlic in 1 tablespoon extra-virgin olive oil until tender.

Preheat oven to 350 degrees. In a large bowl, combine ground turkey, carrots, mashed garbanzo beans, garlic, eggs, tomato paste, Worcestershire sauce, brown sugar, dill, seasoning salt, and two tablespoons extra-virgin olive oil. (Clean hands work best for mixing.) Grease 9″ × 5″ loaf pan with splash of extra-virgin olive oil. Add turkey mixture to loaf pan and pat flat. Bake on middle rack for 60 minutes. Remove from oven and let cool and set for 20 minutes before serving.

———————————————— ◆◆◆◆ ————————————————

Cabbage Rolls _____

Prep time: about 30 minutes

Cooking time: 60 minutes

Number of servings as described: approximately 4 full meals

Ingredients:

1 medium head cabbage

1½ pounds ground turkey

2 cups garbanzo beans, mashed

1 cup grated carrot

1 onion, diced

3 cloves garlic, minced

2 tablespoons tomato paste

2 large eggs, lightly beaten

2 tablespoons Worcestershire sauce

1 tablespoon brown sugar

2 tablespoons fresh dill

1/2 teaspoon seasoning salt

2 tablespoons extra-virgin olive oil

3 cups tomato juice

Preheat oven to 350 degrees. Set aside tomato juice. In a large bowl, combine all remaining ingredients. (Clean hands work best for mixing.)

Core a medium-sized head of cabbage and submerge in water to soften the leaves. Remove leaves as they become pliable. Fill cabbage leaves with enough filling to complete a roll, placed seam side down in casserole dish. After using all the filling, cover rolls with tomato juice. Bake for one hour and serve hot.

Mussels au Gratin _____

Prep time: about
30 minutes

Cooking time: about
15 minutes

Number of servings
as described: 2
protein servings

Ingredients:

3 dozen mussels

1/2 onion, finely chopped

4 cloves garlic, minced

2 tablespoons dried parsley or 1/2 cup fresh parsley,
    finely chopped

1 cup grated reduced-fat cheddar cheese

1/2 cup grated parmesan cheese

2 tablespoons extra-virgin olive oil

1/2 tablespoon lemon pepper

1 whole lemon cut into wedges

Scrub mussels under cold running water. Discard any that do not close. Remove stringy beards. Add about 1″ of water to a large pot and bring to a boil. Reduce to a medium heat and add mussels. Steam mussels until they open; about 8–10 minutes. Pour steamed mussels into a colander and rinse gently in cold water until they are cool enough to handle. Discard any mussels that have not opened. Break off and discard top shell and transfer mussels onto baking pans or cookie sheets.

Preheat oven to 400 degrees. Heat extra-virgin olive oil over medium heat in a medium skillet. Sauté garlic and onion until onion is tender. Add parsley, cheeses, and lemon juice, stirring constantly. Cook until cheeses are melted and mixture is well blended. Add about 1 teaspoon of cheese mixture to each mussel. Bake at 400 degrees for about 5 minutes. Serve warm with lemon wedges.

————————————————✦✦✦✦✦————————————————

Portobello Chicken _____

Prep time: 2 minutes

Cooking time: 25–30
minutes

Number of servings
as described: 4
protein servings

Ingredients:

4 skinless, boneless chicken breasts

4 tablespoons extra-virgin olive oil

8 tablespoons white wine, divided in half

1 portobello mushroom, sliced thinly and divided
    into four portions

fresh ground pepper to taste

salt to taste

Preheat oven to 350 degrees. Lay breasts flat in a baking pan and place several mushroom slices on top of each chicken breast. Pour one tablespoon each of extra-virgin olive oil and white wine over each chicken breast. Bake on a middle rack for 20–25 minutes or until juice runs clear and meat is no longer pink. Remove cooked chicken from oven. Pour one additional tablespoon of white wine over each breast and let sit for 2 minutes before serving.

Good Morning Kick in the Pants Smoothie

Prep Time: 1 minute

Cook time: less than 1 minute

Number of servings as described: 1 full serving of protein

Ingredients:

1½ cups of skim milk

20 grams vanilla whey protein powder

2 teaspoons instant cocoa mix

2 teaspoons instant coffee

Heat milk in microwave for 50 seconds. Add remaining ingredients and mix thoroughly with a hand blender. And voila—a great breakfast and coffee drink all in one!

Berry Medley Fruit Smoothie

Prep time: 5 minutes

Number of servings as described: 1 full meal

Ingredients:

20 grams vanilla or plain whey protein powder

1 cup skim milk

1 cup ice cubes

1/2 cup low- or nonfat plain yogurt

1/2 cup frozen blueberries

1/2 cup frozen strawberries

1/2 frozen banana

Blend in blender until smooth and creamy.

Banana Mocha Smoothie _____

Prep time: 5 minutes

Number of servings as described: 1 full meal

Ingredients:

20 grams chocolate whey protein powder

1 cup skim milk

1/2 frozen banana

10 oz. cold coffee

1 tablespoon peanut butter

1 cup ice cubes

Blend in blender until smooth and creamy.

————————————————— ,,,,, —————————————————

Tropical Fruit Smoothie _____

Prep time: 5 minutes

Number of servings as described: 1 full meal

Ingredients:

20 grams vanilla whey protein powder

1/2 cup low- or nonfat plain yogurt

1 cup pineapple juice

1/2 frozen banana

1/2 cup frozen mango

1 cup ice cubes

1 teaspoon coconut extract

Blend in blender until smooth.

————————————————— ,,,,, —————————————————

Spicy Smoothie _____

Prep time: 5 minutes

Number of servings as described: 1 full serving of protein

Ingredients:

20 grams vanilla whey protein powder

1/2 cup milk

1/2 cup brewed chai tea, chilled

1/2 teaspoon almond extract

1 cup ice cubes

dash cinnamon

Blend in blender until smooth.

RECIPES FOR WEEKS 5–6

....

Protein Pancakes

Prep time: about
5 minutes

Cooking time: about
3 minutes/pancake

Number of servings
as described: about 2
protein servings
(about 6 pancakes)

Ingredients:
40 grams vanilla whey protein
2 cups water
3/4 cup dry pancake mix
6 teaspoons extra-virgin olive oil
maple syrup

In a medium-sized bowl, combine all ingredients and whisk well, making sure there are no clumps of batter remaining. Heat one teaspoon of extra-virgin olive oil in a medium skillet over medium heat. Pour 1/2 cup of batter into skillet. Cook pancake until bottom surface is lightly browned and batter is firm throughout. Flip and cook until opposite surface is lightly browned. Remove cooked pancake, add another teaspoon of olive oil to skillet, and repeat procedure for remaining batter. Serve with maple syrup; up to 2 tablespoons per 3 pancakes.

Chicken Nuggets

Prep time: about
5 minutes

Cooking time: about
10 minutes

Number of servings
as described: about
2 protein servings

Ingredients:

3/4 lb. skinless boneless chicken breasts cut
    into $1^1/_2''$ chunks
1/3 cup wheat-free baking mix
1 teaspoon dry parsley flakes
1 lemon cut into wedges
extra-virgin olive oil

Combine baking mix and parsley in a medium-sized bowl. Roll raw chicken chunks in dry baking mix, breading all surfaces. In a large skillet or saucepan, heat about 1/8″ extra-virgin olive oil over low-medium heat. Lay chicken flat in hot oil and fry until bottom surface is golden brown and chicken is nearly cooked. Flip each piece of chicken and fry opposite surface until golden brown. Make sure chicken nuggets are cooked through; insides should be white with no pink remaining. Serve hot with lemon wedges.

❯❯❯❯❯

Chicken Quesadillas

Prep time: about 10
minutes

Cooking time:
about 15 minutes

Number of servings
as described:
approximately 2
servings of protein
plus 1 serving of
vegetables

Ingredients:

3/4 lb. skinless boneless chicken breast cut into 2" slices
2 cloves garlic, minced
1 cup reduced-fat cheddar cheese, grated, divided
1 avocado, peeled, pitted, and sliced
4 tablespoons nonfat sour cream, divided
4 tablespoons extra-virgin olive oil
2 medium soft-shell flour tortillas
salsa

Heat 2 tablespoons extra-virgin olive oil in a medium skillet over medium heat. Add chicken and garlic. Cook until chicken is tender and lightly browned on all sides, stirring frequently. Remove chicken from skillet and set aside. Add another tablespoon of olive oil to skillet. Lay one tortilla flat, heat for a few seconds in olive oil, and flip. Sprinkle half of cheese onto burrito and top with half of warm chicken. Reduce heat to low-medium, cover, and cook until cheese is melted and tortilla is crunchy. Transfer tortilla to a plate and add half of avocado, 2 tablespoons sour cream, and salsa to taste. Repeat procedure with second tortilla.

Tropical Spicy Shrimp

Prep time: about 15 minutes

Cooking time: about 10 minutes

Number of servings as described: about 3 full meals

Ingredients:

1 lb. raw prawns, peeled and deveined

2 red bell peppers, gutted and sliced

1 mango, chopped into bite-size pieces

1 tablespoon extra-virgin olive oil

1 teaspoon anise seeds

1 clove garlic, minced

1 small onion, diced

2 tablespoons fresh grated ginger

Sauce Ingredients:

2 tablespoons Thai sweet chili sauce

1 tablespoon ketchup

2 tablespoons cider vinegar

1/2 cup water

1 teaspoon cornstarch

In a small bowl, combine and mix sauce ingredients. Heat extra-virgin olive oil in a large skillet or wok on medium heat. Sprinkle anise seeds over oil. Crush seeds slightly into oil with a spoon; allow to warm for 1 or 2 minutes until aromatic. Increase heat to medium high. Add garlic, onions, and ginger, stir frying until slightly tender. Add prawns and stir fry until prawns are just turning pink. Add peppers and mango and stir fry for about 1 minute, allowing to cook yet remain firm. Quickly pour in sauce and heat throughout. Enjoy!

—————————————————— ❥❥❥❥❥ ——————————————————

No Fear Portable Burritos

Prep time: about 20 minutes

Cooking time: about 10 minutes

Number of servings as described: approximately 10 servings of protein (10 burritos)

Ingredients:

2½ lbs. ground turkey or extra lean ground beef

1/2 cup spaghetti sauce

8 oz. salsa

2 oz. burrito seasoning

4 cups grated low-fat cheddar cheese

30 oz. can nonfat refried beans

2–3 tablespoons hot sauce

10 medium soft-shell flour tortillas

Brown ground turkey or beef in saucepan. Pour fat off. Combine remaining ingredients and mix well. Wrap mixture in burrito shells and heat in oven at 350 degrees for 10 minutes. Burritos may also be frozen for later consumption. Simply reheat frozen burritos in oven at 350 degrees for 20 minutes.

◆◆◆◆◆

Grilled Salmon

Prep time: 10 minutes, plus one hour to marinate

Cooking time: about 20 minutes

Number of servings as described: approximately 4 servings of protein

Ingredients:
1$\frac{1}{2}$ lbs. salmon fillet

Marinade Ingredients:
1 cup low-sodium soy sauce
2 tablespoons extra-virgin olive oil
lemon juice from two lemons
2 cloves garlic, minced
1/4 teaspoon fresh ground pepper
1/4 teaspoon basil
2 tablespoons brown sugar

In a small bowl, combine marinade ingredients and mix well. Place salmon fillet in a large bowl and add marinade. If necessary, additional soy sauce may be added so that liquid covers fish. Refrigerate for 1 hour.

Preheat oven to 350 degrees. Place salmon and marinade in roasting pan or casserole dish. Cover and bake for 20–25 minutes or until salmon flakes easily when pressed with a fork. Serve over brown rice and/or grilled vegetables.

◆◆◆◆◆

Lite Lasagna

Prep time: about 20 minutes

Cooking time: 30 minutes

Number of servings as described: approximately 12 servings of protein

Ingredients:
2$\frac{1}{2}$ lbs. ground turkey or extra lean ground beef
6 cloves garlic
5 lasagna noodles, precooked
3 cups spaghetti sauce
2 cups grated reduced-fat mozzarella cheese (about 10 oz.)
2 cups grated reduced-fat cheddar cheese (about 10 oz.)
16 oz. fat-free ricotta cheese
6 egg whites

4 tablespoons grated Parmesan cheese
extra-virgin olive oil to grease casserole dish

Preheat oven to 350 degrees. Brown ground turkey or beef with garlic in a large skillet over medium heat. Pour off fat. Combine cooked turkey or beef with spaghetti sauce and mix well. In a separate bowl, combine ricotta cheese with raw egg whites and beat well. Add the following layers to lightly greased 9″ x 12″ casserole dish (bottom up):

1. half of ground meat/sauce mixture
2. half of grated mozzarella cheese
3. half of grated cheddar cheese
4. ricotta cheese/egg white mixture
5. lasagna noodles
6. second half of ground meat/sauce mixture
7. second half of grated mozzarella cheese
8. second half of grated cheddar cheese
9. top with grated Parmesan cheese

Bake at 350 degrees on a middle rack for 30 minutes. Set aside to cool and set for 20 minutes before serving.

————————————————— ,,,,, —————————————————

Thin Crust Sausage and Garlic Pizza _____

Prep time: about 30 minutes

Cooking time: about 15 minutes

Servings as described: approximately 4 servings of protein

Crust Ingredients:
 1 egg
 1/2 cup dry instant oatmeal
 1/2–3/4 cup whole wheat flour
 1/2 pkg. fast-rising yeast
 1/2 tablespoon extra-virgin olive oil

Topping Ingredients:
 1 package (4 links) low-fat smoked (turkey & chicken) Italian sausage, sliced into 1/8″ rounds
 4 white mushrooms, thinly sliced
 1/2 onion, thinly sliced
 1/2 green pepper, thinly sliced
 1 cup spaghetti sauce
 1 cup reduced-fat mozzarella cheese, grated

1 cup reduced-fat cheddar cheese, grated

4 tablespoons grated Parmesan cheese

3 cloves garlic, minced

1/2 tablespoon extra-virgin olive oil

In a mixing bowl, combine egg and oatmeal. Dissolve 1/2 packet dry yeast in 1/4 cup warm water and add to mixture. Beat well, adding flour a little at a time until dough is firm, not sticky. Set aside to rise for 15 minutes.

Preheat oven to 400 degrees. Grease 12" pizza pan with extra-virgin olive oil. Roll dough flat onto pan.

Sauté minced garlic in small saucepan using extra-virgin olive oil. Stir sautéed garlic into spaghetti sauce. Spread sauce evenly over dough. Sprinkle reduced fat cheeses over sauce. Top with sliced sausage, vegetables, and parmesan cheese. Bake on middle rack at 400 degrees for 15 minutes or until crust starts to brown.

———————————————— ◆◆◆◆◆ ————————————————

5-Minute Personal Pepperoni Pizza

Prep time: about 5 minutes

Cooking time: about 10 minutes

Number of servings as described: approximately 1 serving of protein

Ingredients:

1 link low-fat (turkey & chicken) smoked Italian sausage, sliced into 1/8" rounds

1/2 cup reduced fat grated cheddar and/or mozzarella cheese

3 tablespoons tomato sauce

1 tablespoon extra-virgin olive oil

1 medium soft-shell flour tortilla

Using a medium skillet over medium heat, sauté smoked sausage rounds in extra-virgin olive oil for about five minutes, stirring frequently. Remove sausage from skillet, leaving olive oil and juices in pan. Reduce to low-medium heat and lay tortilla flat, heat for a few seconds, and flip. Spread spaghetti sauce onto tortilla. Then sprinkle cheese over tomato sauce and lay sausage rounds on top of cheese. Cover and cook until cheese is melted and tortilla is crispy.

References

CHAPTER 1
The Un-Diet

Cordain L. The nutritional characteristics of a contemporary diet based upon Paleolithic food groups. Journal of the American Neutraceutical Association 5(3) (2002).

———. Cereal grains: Humanity's double-edged sword. World Review of Nutrition and Dietetics 84 (1999): 19–73.

Cordain L, Brand-Miller J, Eaton SB, Mann N, Holt SH, Speth JD. Plant-animal subsistence ratios and macronutrient energy estimations in worldwide hunter-gatherer diets. American Journal of Clinical Nutrition 71(3) (Mar 2000): 682–92.

Cordain L, Eaton SB, Brand-Miller J, Mann N, Hill K. The paradoxical nature of hunter-gatherer diets: meat-based, yet non-atherogenic. European Journal of Clinical Nutrition 56 Suppl 1 (2002): S42–S52.

Cordain L, Eaton SB, Sebastian A, Mann N, Lindeberg S, Watkins BA, O'Keefe JH, Brand-Miller B, Origins and evolution of the Western diet: Health implications for the 21st century. American Journal of Clinical Nutrition 81 (2005): 341–54.

Cordain L, Gotshall RW, Eaton SB. Evolutionary Aspects of Exercise. Nutrition and fitness: Evolutionary aspects. Children's Health. Programs and Policies. World Review of Nutrition and Dietetics. Basel, Karger. 81 (1997): 49–60.

Daniel M, Rowley KG, McDermott R, Mylvaganam A, O'Dea K. Diabetes incidence in an Australian aboriginal population: An 8-year follow-up study. Diabetes Care 22 (1999): 1993–8.

Easton SB, Konner M. Stone Agers in the fast lane: Chronic degenerative diseases in evolutionary perspective. American Journal of Medicine 84 (1988): 739–49.

Ebbesson SO, Schraer CD, Risica PM, et al. Diabetes and impaired glucose tolerance in three Alaskan Eskimo populations: The Alaska Siberia Project. Diabetes Care 21 (1998): 563–9.

Fagan BM. *People of the Earth: An introduction to world prehistory*. 7th ed. New York: Lehigh Press, 1992.

Lindberg S, Cordain L, Eaton SB. Biological and clinical potential of a Paleolithic diet. Journal of Nutritional and Environmental Medicine 13(3) (Sept 2003): 149–60.

Mann N. Dietary lean red meat and human evolution. European Journal of Nutrition. 39(2) (Apr 2000): 71–9.

Mann NJ. Paleolithic nutrition: What can we learn from the past? Asia Pacific Journal of Clinical Nutrition 13 Suppl (2004): S17.

O'Keefe JH, Cordain L. Cardiovascular disease resulting from a diet and lifestyle at odds with our Paleolithic genome: How to become a 21st-century hunter-gatherer. Mayo Clinic Proceedings (79) (2004): 101–8.

CHAPTER 2
Protein for Pulverizing Paunch

Agus MSD, Swain JF, Larson CL, Eckert EA, and Ludwig DS. Dietary composition and physiologic adaptations to energy restriction. American Journal of Clinical Nutrition 71(4) (Apr 2000): 901–7.

Bloomgarden ZT. Diet and diabetes. Diabetes Care 27(11) (2004).

Bonjour JP. Dietary protein: An essential nutrient for bone health. Journal of the American College of Nutrition. 24(90006) (2005): 526S–536S.

Buchholz AC, Schoeller DA. Is a calorie a calorie? American Journal of Clinical Nutrition 79(5) (May 2004): 899S–906S.

Butterfield GE. Whole-body protein utilization in humans. Medicine and Science in Sports and Exercise 19 (1987): S167–S165.

Chernoff R. Protein and older adults. Journal of the American College of Nutrition 23(90006) (2004): 627S–630S.

Cordain L. The nutritional characteristics of a contemporary diet based upon Paleolithic food groups. Journal of the American Neutraceutical Association 5(3) (2002).

Cordain L, Brand-Miller J, Eaton SB, Mann N, Holt SH, Speth JD. Plant-animal subsistence ratios and macronutrient energy estimations in worldwide hunter-gatherer diets. American Journal of Clinical Nutrition 71(3) (Mar 2000): 682–92.

References

Cordain L, Eaton SB, Brand-Miller J, Mann N, Hill K. The paradoxical nature of hunter-gatherer diets: Meat-based, yet non-atherogenic. European Journal of Clinical Nutrition 56, Suppl 1 (2002): S42–S52.

Cordain L, Eaton SB, Sebastian A, Mann N, Lindeberg S, Watkins BA, O'Keefe JH, Brand-Miller B. Origins and evolution of the Western diet: Health implications for the 21st century. American Journal of Clinical Nutrition 81 (2005): 341–54.

Fielding RA, Parkington J. What are the dietary protein requirements of physically active individuals? New evidence on the effects of exercise on protein utilization during post-exercise recovery. Nutrition in Clinical Care 5(4) (July-Aug 2002): 191–6.

Halton TL, Hu FB. The effects of high protein diets on thermogenesis, satiety and weight loss: A critical review. Journal of the American College of Nutrition 23(5) (2004): 373–85.

Johnston, CS. Strategies for healthy weight loss: From vitamin C to the glycemic response. Journal of the American College of Nutrition 24(3) (2005): 158–65.

Johnston CS, Tjonn SL, Swan PD. High-protein, low-fat diets are effective for weight loss and favorably alter biomarkers in healthy adults. Journal of Nutrition 134(3) (Mar 2004): 586–91.

Layman, DK. Protein quantity and quality at levels above the RDA improves adult weight loss. Journal of the American College of Nutrition 23(90006) (2004): 631S–636S.

Layman DK, Evans E, Baum JI, Seyler J, Erickson DJ, Boileau RA. Dietary protein and exercise have additive effects on body composition during weight loss in adult women. Journal of Nutrition 135(8) (Aug 2005): 1903–10.

Lemon, PWR. Factors which appear to affect dietary protein need. Journal of the American College of Nutrition 19(90005) (2000): 513S–521S.

O'Keefe JH, Cordain L. Cardiovascular disease resulting from a diet and lifestyle at odds with our Paleolithic genome: How to become a 21st-century hunter-gatherer. Mayo Clinic Proceedings 79 (2004): 101–8.

Phillips SM, Hartman JW, Wilkinson SB. Dietary protein to support anabolism with resistance exercise in young men. Journal of the American College of Nutrition 24(2) (2005): 134S–139S.

Rennie MJ, Tipton KD. Protein and amino acid metabolism during and after exercise and the effects of nutrition. Annual Review of Nutrition 20 (2000): 457–83.

Stanko RT, Tietze DL, Arch JE. Body composition, nitrogen metabolism, and energy utilization with feeding of mildly restricted (4.2 MJ/D) and severely restricted (2.1 MJ/D) isonitrogenous diets. American Journal of Clinical Nutrition 56(4) (Oct 1992): 636–40.

Street C. High-protein intake—Is it safe? In: Antonio J, Stout JR, eds. Sports Supplements, pp. 311–312. Philadelphia: Lippincott Williams & Wilkins (2001).

CHAPTER 3
Fat for a Fabulous Physique

Ascherio A, Katan MB, Zock PL, Stampfer MJ, Willett WC. Trans fatty acids and coronary heart disease. The New England Journal of Medicine 340(25) (June 24, 1999).

Auer J, Berent R, Lassnig E, Eber B. C-reactive protein and coronary artery disease. Japanese Heart Journal 43(6) (Nov 2002): 607–19.

Aude YW, Agatston AS, Lopez-Jimenez F, Lieberman EH, Marie Almon, Hansen M, Rojas G, Lamas GA, Hennekens CH. The national cholesterol education program diet vs a diet lower in carbohydrates and higher in protein and monounsaturated fat: A randomized trial. Archives of Internal Medicine 164(19) (Oct 25, 2004): 2141–6.

Brehm BJ, Spang SE, Lattin BL, Seeley RJ, Daniels SR, and D'Alessio DA. The role of energy expenditure in the differential weight loss in obese women on low-fat and low-carbohydrate diets. Journal of Clinical Endocrinology and Metabolism 90(3) (Mar 2005): 1475–82.

Canadian Institute for Health Information. Improving the health of Canadians. Ottawa: Canadian Institute for Health Information (2004).

Cordain L. The nutritional characteristics of a contemporary diet based upon Paleolithic food groups. Journal of the American Neutraceutical Association 5(3) (2002).

———. Cereal Grains: Humanity's double-edged sword. World Review of Nutrition and Dietetics 84 (1999): 19–73.

Cordain L, Brand-Miller J, Eaton SB, Mann N, Holt SH, Speth JD. Plant-animal subsistence ratios and macronutrient energy estimations in worldwide hunter-gatherer diets. American Journal of Clinical Nutrition 71(3) (Mar 2000): 682–92.

Cordain L, Eaton SB, Brand-Miller J, Mann N, Hill K. The paradoxical nature of hunter-gatherer diets: meat-based, yet non-atherogenic. European Journal of Clinical Nutrition 56, Suppl 1 (2002): S42–S52.

Cordain L, Eaton SB, Sebastian A, Mann N, Lindeberg S, Watkins BA, O'Keefe JH, Brand-Miller B, Origins and evolution of the Western diet: health implications for the 21st century. American Journal of Clinical Nutrition 81 (2005): 341–54.

Cordain L, Watkins BA, Florant1 GL, Kelher, M, Rogers L, Li Y. Fatty acid analysis of wild ruminant tissues: Evolutionary implications for reducing diet-related chronic disease. European Journal of Clinical Nutrition 56 (2002): 181–91.

References

Eaton B, Eaton III SB, Sinclair AJ, Cordain L, Mannb NJ. Dietary intake of long-chain polyunsaturated fatty acids during the Paleolithic. World Review of Nutrition and Dietetics. Basel, Karger. 83 (1998): 12–23 S.

Enig M. Diet, serum cholesterol and coronary heart disease. In G. Mann, Coronary Heart Disease (1993).

Enig MG and Fallon SW. The oiling of America. *Nexus Magazine* (Dec–Jan 1999; Feb–Mar 1999).

Enig, MG, et al. Dietary fat and cancer trends—A critique. Federation Proceedings 37(9) (July 1978): 2215–2220, FASEB.

Fallon S, Enig, MG., PhD. The great con-ola, Wise Traditions in Food, Farming and the Healing Arts, the quarterly magazine of the Weston A. Price Foundation (Summer 2002).

Flegal KM, Carroll MD, Kuczmarski RJ, Johnson CL. Overweight and obesity in the United States: Prevalence and trends, 1960–1994. International Journal of Obesity Related Metabolic Disorders 22(1) (Jan 1998): 39–47.

Gamba CA, Friedman SM, Rodriguez PN, Macri EV, Vacas MI, Lifshitz F. Metabolic status in growing rats fed isocaloric diets with increased carbohydrate-to-fat ratio. Nutrition 21(2) (Feb 2005): 249–54.

Health Canada. Canadian guidelines for body weight classification in adults (Catalogue H49-179) Ottawa: Health Canada (2003).

Iunis SM, Dyer RA. Dietary canola oil alters hematological indices and blood lipids in neonatal piglets fed formula. *Journal of Nutrition* 129(7) (July 1999): 1261–8.

Khor GL. Dietary fat quality: a nutritional epidemiologist's view. Asia Pacific Journal of Clinical Nutrition 13(Suppl) (Aug 2004): S22.

Kramer JK, Farnworth ER, Thompson BK, Corner AH, Trenholm HL. Reduction of myocardial necrosis in male albino rats by manipulation of dietary fatty acid levels. Lipids 17(5) (1982 May): 372–82.

Kramer JK, Sauer FD, Farnworth ER, Stevenson D, Rock GA. Hematological and lipid changes in newborn piglets fed milk-replacer diets containing erucic acid. Lipids 33(1) (January 1998): 1–10.

Levander OA, Beck MA. Selenium and viral virulence. British Medical Bulletin 55(3) (1999): 528–33.

Lindberg S, Cordain L, Eaton SB. Biological and clinical potential of a Palaeolithic diet. Journal of Nutritional and Environmental Medicine 13(3) (September 2003): 149–60.

Manginas A, Bei E, Chaidaroglou A, Degiannis D, Koniavitou K, Voudris V, Pavlides G, Panagiotakos D, Cokkinos DV. Peripheral levels of matrix metalloproteinase–9, interleukin–6, and C-reactive protein are elevated in patients with acute coronary syndromes: correlations with serum troponin I. Clinical Cardiology 28(4) (Apr 2005): 182–6.

Meckling KA, O'Sullivan C, Saari D. Comparison of a low-fat diet to a low-carbohydrate diet on weight loss, body composition, and risk factors for diabetes and cardiovascular disease in free-living, overweight men and women. Journal of Clinical Endocrinology and Metabolism 89(6) (Jun 2004): 2717–23.

Meksawan K, Pendergast DR, Leddy JJ, Mason M, Horvath PJ, Awad AB. Effect of low and high fat diets on nutrient intakes and selected cardiovascular risk factors in sedentary men and women. Journal of the American College of Nutrition 23(2) (2004): 131–40.

Mullis RM, Blair SN, Aronne LJ, Bier DM, Denke MA, Dietz W, Donato KA, Drewnowski A, French SA, Howard BV, Robinson TN, Swinburn B, Wechsler H. Obesity, a worldwide epidemic related to heart disease and stroke: Group IV: Prevention/Treatment. AHA Conference Proceedings, Prevention Conference VII, *Circulation* 110 (2004): e484–e488. (Copyright 2004 American Heart Association, Inc.)

O'Keefe JH, Cordain L. Cardiovascular disease resulting from a diet and lifestyle at odds with our Paleolithic genome: How to become a 21st-century hunter-gatherer. Mayo Clinic Proceedings 79 (2004): 101–8.

O'Keefe S, Gaskins-Wright S, Wiley V, Chen-Chen I. Level of trans geometrical isomers of essential fatty acids in some unhydrogenated U.S. vegetable oils. Journal of Food Lipids 1 (1994): 165–76.

Ravnskov, U. The questionable role of saturated and polyunsaturated fatty acids in cardiovascular disease. Journal of Clinical Epidemiology 51(6) (1998): 443–60.

Sauer FD, Farnworth ER, Belanger JMR, Kramer JKG, Miller RB, Yamashiro S. Additional vitamin E required in milk replacer diets that contain canola oil. *Nutrition Research* 17(2) (1997): 259–69.

Statement of Senator George McGovern on the Publication of Dietary Goals for the United States. Press Conference, Friday, January 14, (1977, Room 457, Dirksen Office Building).

Vles RO, Bijster GM, Timmer WG. Nutritional evaluation of low-erucic-acid rapeseed oils. Toxicological Aspects of Food Safety, *Archives of Toxicology* Suppl 1 (1978): 23–32.

Volek J, Sharman M, Gomez A, Judelson D, Rubin M, Watson G, Sokmen B, Silvestre R, French D, Kraemer W. Comparison of energy-restricted very low-carbohydrate and low-fat diets on weight loss and body composition in overweight men and women. Nutrition and Metabolism (London) 1(1) (Nov 8, 2004): 13.

CHAPTER 4
Carbohydrates Part I:
Friendly Fire for Burning Fat

Aller R, de Luis DA, Izaola O, La Calle F, del Olmo L, Fernandez L, Arranz T, Hernandez JM. Effect of soluble fiber intake in lipid and glucose levels in healthy subjects: A randomized clinical trial. Diabetes Research and Clinical Practice 65(1) (Jul 2004): 7–11.

Bingham SA, Day NE, Luben R, et al. Dietary fibre in food and protection against colorectal cancer in the European Prospective Investigation into Cancer and Nutrition (EPIC): An observational study, Lancet 361 (2003): 1496–1501.

Brown L, Rosner B, Willett WW, Sacks FM. Cholesterol-lowering effects of dietary fiber: A meta-analysis. American Journal of Clinical Nutrition 69 (1999): 30–42.

Cordain L. The nutritional characteristics of a contemporary diet based upon Paleolithic food groups. Journal of the American Neutraceutical Association 5(3) (2002).

Cordain L, Eaton SB, Brand-Miller J, Mann N, Hill K. The paradoxical nature of hunter-gatherer diets: Meat-based, yet non-atherogenic. European Journal of Clinical Nutrition 56, Suppl 1 (2002): S42–S52.

Cordain L, Eaton SB, Sebastian A, Mann N, Lindeberg S, Watkins BA, O'Keefe JH, Brand-Miller B. Origins and evolution of the Western diet: Health implications for the 21st century. American Journal of Clinical Nutrition 81 (2005): 341–54.

Cordain L, Brand-Miller J, Eaton SB, Mann N, Holt SH, Speth JD. Plant-animal subsistence ratios and macronutrient energy estimations in worldwide hunter-gatherer diets. American Journal of Clinical Nutrition 71(3) (Mar 2000): 682–92.

Higgins JA. Resistant starch: Metabolic effects and potential health benefits. Journal of AOAC International 87 (2004): 761–7.

Jensen C, Haskell W, Whittam J. Long-term effects of water-soluble dietary fiber in the management of hypercholesterolemia in healthy men and women. American Journal of Cardiology 79 (1997): 34–7.

McIntosh M, Miller C. A diet containing food rich in soluble and insoluble fiber improves glycemic control and reduces hyperlipidemia among patients with type 2 diabetes mellitus. Nutrition Reviews (Feb 2001).

Pereira MA, O'Reilly E, Augustsson K, et al. Dietary fiber and risk of coronary heart disease: A pooled analysis of cohort studies. Archives of Internal Medicine 164 (2004): 370–76.

Peters U, Sinha R, Chatterjee N, et al. Dietary fibre and colorectal adenoma in a colorectal cancer study detection programme. Lancet 361 (2003): 1491–5.

Tiwary CM, Ward JA, Jackson BA. Effect of pectin on satiety in healthy US Army adults. Journal of the American College of Nutrition 16(5) (Oct 1997): 423–8.

Wakai K, Hirose K, Matsuo K, Ito H, Kuriki K, Suzuki T, Kato T, Hirai T, Kanemitsu Y, Tajima K. Dietary risk factors for colon and rectal cancers: a comparative case-control study. Journal of Epidemiology 16(3) (May 2006): 125–35.

CHAPTER 5
Carbohydrates Part II:
Glycemic Response and the Bane of the Grain

Aller R, de Luis DA, Izaola O, La Calle F, del Olmo L, Fernandez L, Arranz T, Hernandez JM. Effect of soluble fiber intake in lipid and glucose levels in healthy subjects: A randomized clinical trial. Diabetes Research and Clinical Practice 65(1) (Jul 2004): 7–11.

Chiu CJ, Hubbard LD, Armstrong J, Rogers G, Jacques PF, Chylack LT Jr, Hankinson SE, Willett WC, Taylor A. Dietary glycemic index and carbohydrate in relation to early age-related macular degeneration. American Journal of Clinical Nutrition. 83(4) (Apr 2006): 880–86.

Cordain L. The nutritional characteristics of a contemporary diet based upon Paleolithic food groups. Journal of the American Neutraceutical Association 5(3) (2002).

Cordain, L. Cereal grains: Humanity's double-edged sword. World Review of Nutrition and Dietetics 84 (1999): 19–73.

Cordain L, Eaton SB, Brand-Miller J, Mann N, Hill K. The paradoxical nature of hunter-gatherer diets: Meat-based, yet non-atherogenic. European Journal of Clinical Nutrition 56 Suppl 1 (2002): S42–S52.

Cordain L, Eaton SB, Sebastian A, Mann N, Lindeberg S, Watkins BA, O'Keefe JH, Brand-Miller B. Origins and evolution of the Western diet: Health implications for the 21st century. American Journal of Clinical Nutrition 81 (2005): 341–54.

Feinman RD, Fine EJ. "A calorie is a calorie" violates the second law of thermodynamics. Nutrition Journal 3 (2004): 9.

Johnston, CS. Strategies for healthy weight loss: From vitamin C to the glycemic response. Journal of the American College of Nutrition 24(3) (2005): 158–65.

Liu S, Willett WC, Stampfer MJ, et al. A prospective study of dietary glycemic load, carbohydrate intake, and risk of coronary heart disease in US women. American Journal of Clinical Nutrition 71 (2000): 1455–61.

Lofgren IE, Herron KL, West KL, Zern TL, Brownbill RA, Ilich JZ, Koo SI, Fernandez ML. Weight loss favorably modifies anthropometrics and reverses the metabolic syndrome in premenopausal women. Journal of the American College of Nutrition 24(6) (2005): 486–93.

Ma Y, Li Y, Chiriboga DE, Olendzki BC, Hebert JR, Li W, Leung K, Hafner AR, Ockene IS. Association between carbohydrate intake and serum lipids. Journal of the American College of Nutrition 25(2) (2006): 155–63.

McIntosh M, Miller C. A diet containing food rich in soluble and insoluble fiber improves glycemic control and reduces hyperlipidemia among patients with type 2 diabetes mellitus. Nutrition Reviews 59(2)(Feb 2001): 52–5.

McKeown NM, Meigs JB, Liu S, Saltzman E, Wilson PW, Jacques PF. Carbohydrate nutrition, insulin resistance, and the prevalence of the metabolic syndrome in the Framingham Offspring Cohort. Diabetes Care 27 (2004): 538–46.

McKeown NM, Meigs JB, Liu S, Wilson PW, Jacques PF. Whole-grain intake is favorably associated with metabolic risk factors for type 2 diabetes and cardiovascular disease in the Framingham Offspring Study. American Journal of Clinical Nutrition 76 (2002): 390–98.

McMillan-Price J, Petocz P, Atkinson F, O'Neill K, Samman S, Steinbeck K, Caterson I, Brand-Miller J. Comparison of 4 diets of varying glycemic load on weight loss and cardiovascular risk reduction in overweight and obese young adults: A randomized controlled trial. Archives of Internal Medicine 166(14) (Jul 24, 2006): 1466–75.

Pereira MA, O'Reilly E, Augustsson K, et al. Dietary fiber and risk of coronary heart disease: A pooled analysis of cohort studies. Archives of Internal Medicine 164 (2004): 370–76.

Pereira MA, Swain J, Goldfine AB, Rifai N, Ludwig DS. Effects of a low-glycemic load diet on resting energy expenditure and heart disease risk factors during weight loss. Journal of the American Medical Association 292 (2004): 2482–2490.

Schulze MB, Liu S, Rimm EB, Manson JE, Willett WC, Hu FB. Glycemic index, glycemic load, and dietary fiber intake and incidence of type 2 diabetes in younger and middle-aged women. American Journal of Clinical Nutrition 80 (2004): 348–56.

Steyn NP, Mann J, Bennett PH, Temple N, Zimmet P, Tuomilehto J, Lindstrom J, Louheranta A. Diet, nutrition and the prevention of type 2 diabetes. Public Health Nutrition 7(1A) (Feb 2004): 147–65.

Van Dam RM, Willett WC, Manson JE, Hu FB. The relationship between overweight in adolescence and premature death in women. Annals of Internal Medicine 145(2) (Jul 18, 2006): 91–7.

CHAPTER 6
Micronutrients that Keep You
Lean and Wrinkle-Free

Aas V, Rokling-Andersen MH, Kase ET, Thoresen GH, Rustan AC. Eicosapentaenoic acid (20: 5 n–3) increases fatty acid and glucose uptake in cultured human skeletal muscle cells. Journal of Lipid Research 47(2) (Feb 2006): 366–74.

Ahsan SK. Metabolism of magnesium in health and disease. Journal of the Indian Medical Association 95(9) (Sep 1997): 507–10.

Annual Meeting of the North American Association for the Study of Obesity Abstract #249-P (2004).

Black HS, Rhodes LE. The potential of omega-3 fatty acids in the prevention of non-melanoma skin cancer. Cancer Detection and Prevention 30(3) (2006): 224–32.

Brooks BM, Rajeshwari R, Nicklas TA, Yang SJ, Berenson GS. Association of calcium intake, dairy product consumption with overweight status in young adults (1995–1996): The Bogalusa Heart Study. Journal of the American College of Nutrition 25(6) (Dec 2006): 523–32.

Calon F, Lim GP, Yang F, Morihara T, Teter B, Ubeda O, Rostaing P, Triller A, Salem N Jr, Ashe KH, Frautschy SA, Cole GM. Docosahexaenoic acid protects from dendritic pathology in an Alzheimer's disease mouse model. Neuron 43(5) (Sep 2, 2004): 633–45.

Cappuccio FP. Dietary prevention of osteoporosis: are we ignoring the evidence? American Journal of Clinical Nutrition 63(5) (May 1996): 787–8.

Cappuccio FP, Kalaitzidis R, Duneclift S, Eastwood JB. Unravelling the links between calcium excretion, salt intake, hypertension, kidney stones and bone metabolism. Journal of Nephrology 13(3) (May–Jun 2000): 169–77.

Carbone LD, Barrow KD, Bush AJ, Boatright MD, Michelson JA, Pitts KA, Pintea VN, Kang AH, Watsky MA. Effects of a low sodium diet on bone metabolism. Journal of Bone and Mineral Metabolism 23(6) (2005): 506–13.

Carpenter TO, Delucia MC, Zhang JH, Bejnerowicz G, Tartamella L, Dziura J, Petersen KF, Befroy D, Cohen D. A randomized controlled study of effects of dietary magnesium oxide supplementation on bone mineral content in healthy girls. Journal of Clinical Endocrinology and Metabolism 91(12) (Dec 2006): 4822–72.

Chambers EC, Heshka S, Gallagher D, Wang J, Pi-Sunyer FX, Pierson RN Jr. Serum magnesium and type-2 diabetes in African Americans and Hispanics: A New York cohort. Journal of the American College of Nutrition 25(6) (Dec 2006): 509–13.

Cole GM, Lim GP, Yang F, Teter B, Begum A, Ma Q, Harris-White ME, Frautschy SA. Prevention of Alzheimer's disease: Omega-3 fatty acid and phenolic anti-oxidant interventions. Neurobiology of Aging 26 Suppl 1 (Dec 2005): 133–6.

Cordain L, Gotshall RW, Eaton SB. Evolutionary Aspects of Exercise. Nutrition and Fitness: Evolutionary Aspects. Children's Health. Programs and Policies. World Review of Nutrition and Dietetics 81 (1997): 49–60.

Cummings NK, James AP, Soares MJ. The acute effects of different sources of dietary calcium on postprandial energy metabolism. British Journal of Nutrition 96(1) (Jul 2006): 138–44.

Curtis CL, Rees SG, Cramp J, Flannery CR, Hughes CE, Little CB, Williams R, Wilson C, Dent CM, Harwood JL, Caterson B. Effects of n–3 fatty acids on cartilage metabolism. Proceedings of the Nutrition Society 61(3) (Aug 2002): 381–9.

Davis DR, Epp MD, Riordan HD. Changes in USDA food composition data for 43 garden crops, 1950 to 1999. Journal of the American College of Nutrition 23 (2004): 669–82.

Dean BB, Borenstein JE, Henning JM, Knight K, Merz CN. Can change in high-density lipoprotein cholesterol levels reduce cardiovascular risk? American Heart Journal 147(6) (Jun 2004): 966–76.

Delarue J, LeFoll C, Corporeau C, Lucas D. N–3 long chain polyunsaturated fatty acids: a nutritional tool to prevent insulin resistance associated to type 2 diabetes and obesity? Reproduction Nutrition Development (May–Jun 2004) 44(3): 289–99.

Devine A, Criddle RA, Dick IM, Kerr DA, Prince RL. A longitudinal study of the effect of sodium and calcium intakes on regional bone density in postmenopausal women. American Journal of Clinical Nutrition 62(4) (Oct 1995): 740–45.

Dos Santos LC, Martini LA, Cintra Ide P, Fisberg M. Relationship between calcium intake and body mass index in adolescents. Archivos Latinoamericanos De Nutricion 55(4) (Dec 2005): 345–9.

Duncan AM. The role of nutrition in the prevention of breast cancer. AACN Clinical Issues 15(1) (Jan–Mar 2004): 119–35.

Ergas D, Eilat E, Mendlovic S, Sthoeger ZM. n–3 fatty acids and the immune system in autoimmunity. Israel Medical Association Journal 4(1) (Jan 2002): 34–8.

Farvid MS, Jalali M, Siassi F, Saadat N, Hosseini M. The Impact of Vitamins and/or Mineral Supplementation on Blood Pressure in Type 2 Diabetes. Journal of the American College of Nutrition 23(3) (2004): 272–9.

Flachs P, Horakova O, Brauner P, Rossmeisl M, Pecina P, Franssen-van Hal N, Ruzickova J, Sponarova J, Drahota Z, Vlcek C, Keijer J, Houstek J, Kopecky J. Polyunsaturated fatty acids of marine origin upregulate mitochondrial biogenesis and induce beta-oxidation in white fat. Diabetologia 48(11) (Nov 2005): 2365–75.

Fulgoni III VL, Huth PJ, DiRienzo DB, Miller GD. Determination of the optimal number of dairy servings to ensure a low prevalence of inadequate calcium intake in Americans. Journal of the American College of Nutrition 23(6) (2004): 651–9.

Gonzalez AJ, White E, Kristal A, Littman AJ. Calcium intake and 10-year weight change in middle-aged adults. Journal of the American Dietetic Association 106(7) (Jul 2006): 1066–73.

Heaney RP. Low calcium intake among African Americans: Effects on bones and body weight. Journal of Nutrition 136(4) (Apr 2006): 1095–8.

———. Role of dietary sodium in osteoporosis. Journal of the American College of Nutrition 25(90003) (2006): 271S–276S.

Heaney RP, Weaver CM. Newer perspectives on calcium nutrition and bone quality. Journal of the American College of Nutrition 24(90006) (2005): 574S–581S.

Hercberg S, Galan P, Preziosi P, Bertrais S, Mennen L, Malvy D, Roussel AM, Favier A, Briancon S. The SU.VI.MAX Study: A randomized, placebo-controlled trial of the health effects of antioxidant vitamins and minerals. Archives of Internal Medicine 164(21) (Nov 22, 2004): 2335–42.

Hsieh ST, Sano H, Saito K, Kubota Y, Yokoyama M. Magnesium supplementation prevents the development of alcohol-induced hypertension. Hypertension 19(2) (Feb 1992): 175–82.

Jacobs ET, Martinez ME, Alberts DS. Research and public health implications of the intricate relationship between calcium and vitamin D in the prevention of colorectal neoplasia. Journal of the National Cancer Institute 95(23) (Dec 3, 2003): 1736–7.

James MJ, Cleland LG. Dietary n–3 fatty acids and therapy for rheumatoid arthritis. Seminars in Arthritis and Rheumatism 27(2) (Oct 1997): 85–97. Review.

James MJ, Proudman SM, Cleland LG. Dietary n–3 fats as adjunctive therapy in a prototypic inflammatory disease: issues and obstacles for use in rheumatoid arthritis. Prostaglandins Leukotrienes and Essential Fatty Acids 68(6) (Jun 2003): 399–405.

Johnson EJ, Schaefer EJ. Potential role of dietary n–3 fatty acids in the prevention of dementia and macular degeneration. American Journal of Clinical Nutrition 83(6 Suppl) (Jun 2006): 1494S–1498S.

Johnston, CS. Strategies for healthy weight loss: From vitamin C to the glycemic response. Journal of the American College of Nutrition 24(3) (2005): 158–65.

Kalmijn S. Fatty acid intake and the risk of dementia and cognitive decline: a review of clinical and epidemiological studies. Journal of Nutrition Health Aging 4(4) (2000): 202–7.

Karppanen H, Mervaala E. Sodium intake and hypertension. Progress in Cardiovascular Diseases 49(2) (Sep–Oct 2006): 59–75. Review.

Kim HH, Cho S, Lee S, Kim KH, Cho KH, Eun HC, Chung JH. Photoprotective and anti-skin-aging effects of eicosapentaenoic acid in human skin in vivo. Journal of Lipid Research 47(5) (May 2006): 921–30.

Kim HH, Shin CM, Park CH, Kim KH, Cho KH, Eun HC, Chung JH. Eicosapentaenoic acid inhibits UV-induced MMP–1 expression in human dermal fibroblasts. Journal of Lipid Research 46(8) (Aug 2005): 1712–20.

Kitchin B, Morgan SL. Not just calcium and vitamin D: Other nutritional considerations in osteoporosis. Current Rheumatological Reports 9(1) (Feb 2007): 85–92.

Kousa A, Havulinna AS, Moltchanova E, Taskinen O, Nikkarinen M, Eriksson J, Karvonen M. Calcium:Magnesium ratio in local groundwater and incidence of acute myocardial infarction among males in rural Finland. Environmental Health Perspectives 114(5) (May 2006): 730–34.

Littlefield NA, Hass BS. Is the RDA for magnesium too low? From the 1996 FDA Science Forum. Abstract. NCTR, FDA, Jefferson AR 72079.

Logan AC. Omega-3 fatty acids and acne. Archives of Dermatology 139(7) (Jul 2003): 941–2; author reply 942–3.

Lovelace HY, Barr SI. Diagnosis, symptoms, and calcium intakes of individuals with self-reported lactose intolerance. Journal of the American College of Nutrition 24(1) (2005): 51–7.

Macdonald A. Omega–3 fatty acids as adjunctive therapy in Crohn's disease. Gastroenterology Nursing 29(4) (Jul–Aug 2006): 295–301; quiz 302–3.

MacLean CH, Mojica WA, Newberry SJ, Pencharz J, Garland RH, Tu W, Hilton LG, Gralnek IM, Rhodes S, Khanna P, Morton SC. Systematic review of the effects of n–3 fatty acids in inflammatory bowel disease. American Journal of Clinical Nutrition 82(3) (Sep 2005): 611–19.

Mazza M, Pomponi M, Janiri L, Bria P, Mazza S. Omega-3 fatty acids and antioxidants in neurological and psychiatric diseases: An overview. Progress in Neuro-Psychopharmacology and Biological Psychiatry 31(4) (May 2007): 974.

Mickleborough TD, Rundell KW. Dietary polyunsaturated fatty acids in asthma- and exercise-induced bronchoconstriction. European Journal of Clinical Nutrition 59(12) (Dec 2005): 1335–46.

References

Morris MC, Evans DA, Bienas JL, Tangney CC, Bennett DA, Wilson RS, Aggarwal N, Schneider J. Consumption of fish and n–3 fatty acids and risk of incident Alzheimer disease. Archives of Neurology 60 (2003): 940–46.

Murakami K, Okubo H, Sasaki S. No relation between intakes of calcium and dairy products and body mass index in Japanese women aged 18 to 20 y. Nutrition 22(5) (May 2006): 490–95.

Matsuzaki H. Prevention of osteoporosis by foods and dietary supplements. Magnesium and bone metabolism. Clinical Calcium 16(10) (Oct 2006): 1655–60.

Nettleton JA, Katz R. n–3 long-chain polyunsaturated fatty acids in type 2 diabetes: A review. Journal of the American Dietetic Association 105(3) (Mar 2005): 428–40.

Nordin BE, Need AG, Morris HA, Horowitz M. The nature and significance of the relationship between urinary sodium and urinary calcium in women. Journal of Nutrition 123(9) (Sep 1993): 1615–22.

Olatunji LA, Soladoye AO. Increased magnesium intake prevents hyperlipidemia and insulin resistance and reduces lipid peroxidation in fructose-fed rats. Pathophysiology 14(1) (May 2007): 11–15.

Palacios C. The role of nutrients in bone health, from A to Z. CRC Critical Reviews in Food Science and Nutrition 46(8) (2006): 621–8. Review.

Pokan R, Hofmann P, von Duvillard SP, Smekal G, Wonisch M, Lettner K, Schmid P, Shechter M, Silver B, Bachl N. Oral magnesium therapy, exercise heart rate, exercise tolerance, and myocardial function in coronary artery disease patients. British Journal of Sports Medicine 40(9) (Sep 2006): 773–8.

Rajpathak SN, Rimm EB, Rosner B, Willett WC, Hu FB. Calcium and dairy intakes in relation to long-term weight gain in US men. American Journal of Clinical Nutrition 83(3) (Mar 2006): 559–66.

Rayssiguier Y, Gueux E, Nowacki W, Rock E, Mazur A. High fructose consumption combined with low dietary magnesium intake may increase the incidence of the metabolic syndrome by inducing inflammation. Magnesium Research 19(4) (Dec 2006): 237–43. Review.

Reid IR. Effects of calcium supplementation on circulating lipids: Potential pharmacoeconomic implications. Drugs Aging 21(1) (2004): 7–17.

Reid IR, Mason B, Horne A, Ames R, Clearwater J, Bava U, Orr-Walker B, Wu F, Evans MC, Gamble GD. Effects of calcium supplementation on serum lipid concentrations in normal older women: A randomized controlled trial. American Journal of Medicine 112(5) (Apr 1, 2002): 343–7.

Romieu I, Téllez-Rojo MM, Lazo M, Manzano-Patiño A, Cortez-Lugo M, Julien P, Bélanger MC, Hernandez-Avila M, Holguin F. Omega-3 fatty acid prevents heart rate variability reductions associated with particulate matter. American Journal of Respiratory and Critical Care Medicine 172 (Dec 2005): 1534–40.

Roynette CE, Calder PC, Dupertuis YM, Pichard C. n–3 polyunsaturated fatty acids and colon cancer prevention. Clinical Nutrition 23(2) (Apr 2004): 139–51.

Rubenowitz E, Axelsson G, Rylander R. Magnesium in drinking water and death from acute myocardial infarction. American Journal of Epidemiology 143(5) (Mar 1, 1996): 456–62.

Rumawas ME, McKeown NM, Rogers G, Meigs JB, Wilson PW, Jacques PF. Magnesium intake is related to improved insulin homeostasis in the Framingham offspring cohort. Journal of the American College of Nutrition 25(6) (Dec 2006): 486–92.

Russo BG. Dairy foods, dietary calcium and obesity: A short review of the evidence. Nutrition Metabolism and Cardiovascular Diseases 16(6) (Sep 2006): 445–51.

Ryder KM, Shorr RI, Bush AJ, Kritchevsky SB, Harris T, Stone K, Cauley J, Tylavsky FA. Magnesium intake from food and supplements is associated with bone mineral density in healthy older white subjects. Journal of the American Geriatric Society 53(11) (Nov 2005): 1875–80.

Saugstad LF. Are neurodegenerative disorder and psychotic manifestations avoidable brain dysfunctions with adequate dietary omega-3? Nutrition and Health 18(2) (2006): 89–101.

Schulze MB, Schulz M, Heidemann C, Schienkiewitz A, Hoffmann K, Boeing H. Fiber and magnesium intake and incidence of type 2 diabetes: A prospective study and meta-analysis. Archives of Internal Medicine 167(9) (May 14, 2007): 956–65.

Shechter M, Shechter A. Magnesium and myocardial infarction. Clinical Calcium 15(11) (Nov 2005): 111–15.

Sojka JE, Weaver CM. Magnesium supplementation and osteoporosis. Nutrition Reviews 53(3) (Mar 1995): 71–4.

Song Y, He K, Levitan EB, Manson JE, Liu S. Effects of oral magnesium supplementation on glycaemic control in Type 2 diabetes: a meta-analysis of randomized double-blind controlled trials. Diabetic Medicine 23(10) (Oct 2006): 1050–56.

Song Y, Li TY, van Dam RM, Manson JE, Hu FB. Magnesium intake and plasma concentrations of markers of systemic inflammation and endothelial dysfunction in women. American Journal of Clinical Nutrition 85(4) (Apr 2007): 1068–74.

Song Y, Sesso HD, Manson JE, Cook NR, Buring JE, Liu S. Dietary magnesium intake and risk of incident hypertension among middle-aged and older US women in a 10-year follow-up study. American Journal of Cardiology 98(12) (Dec 15, 2006): 1616–21.

Stendig-Lindberg G, Tepper R, Leichter I. Trabecular bone density in a two year controlled trial of per oral magnesium in osteoporosis. Magnesium Research 6(2) (Jun 1993): 155–63.

Stephensen CB, Kelley DS. The innate immune system: Friend and foe. American Journal of Clinical Nutrition 83(2) (Feb 2006): 187–8.

Sugiyama T, Xie D, Graham-Maar RC, Inoue K, Kobayashi Y, Stettler N. Dietary and lifestyle factors associated with blood pressure among U.S. adolescents. Journal of Adolescent Health 40(2) (Feb 2007): 166–72.

Takezaki T, Inoue M, Kataoka H, Ikeda S, Yoshida M, Ohashi Y, Tajima K, Tominaga S. Diet and lung cancer risk from a 14-year population-based prospective study in Japan: With special reference to fish consumption. Nutrition and Cancer—An International Journal 45(2) (2003): 160–67.

Tomiyama H, Takazawa K, Osa S, Hirose K, Hirai A, Iketani T, Monden M, Sanoyama K, Yamashina A. Do eicosapentaenoic acid supplements attenuate age-related increases in arterial stiffness in patients with dyslipidemia? A preliminary study. Hypertension Research 28(8) (Aug 2005): 651–5.

Trowman R, Dumville JC, Hahn S, Torgerson DJ. A systematic review of the effects of calcium supplementation on body weight. British Journal of Nutrition 95(6) (Jun 2006): 1033–8.

Tujague J, Bastaki M, Holland N, Balmes JR, Tager IB. Antioxidant intake, GSTM1 polymorphism and pulmonary function in healthy young adults. European Respiratory Journal 27(2) (Feb 2006): 282–8.

Uauy R, Dangour AD. Nutrition in brain development and aging: Role of essential fatty acids. Nutrition Reviews 64(5 Pt 2) (May 2006): S24–33; discussion S72–91.

Wakai K, Hirose K, Matsuo K, Ito H, Kuriki K, Suzuki T, Kato T, Hirai T, Kanemitsu Y, Tajima K. Dietary risk factors for colon and rectal cancers: A comparative case-control study. Journal of Epidemiology 16(3) (May 2006): 125–35.

Watson TA, Callister R, Taylor R, David SW, Macdonald-Wicks LK, Garg ML. Antioxidant restriction and oxidative stress in short-duration exhaustive exercise. Medicine and Science in Sports and Exercise 37(1) (Jan 2005): 63–71.

White JR, Campbell RK. Magnesium and diabetes: A review. Annals of Pharmacotherapy 27(6) (Jun 1993): 775–80.

Witteman JC, Grobbee DE, Derkx FH, Bouillon R, de-Bruijn AM, Hofman A. Reduction of blood pressure with oral magnesium supplementation in women with mild to moderate hypertension. American Journal of Clinical Nutrition 60(1) (Jul 1994): 129–35.

Wolters M. The significance of diet and associated factors in psoriasis. Hautarzt 57(11) (Nov 2006): 990–1004.

Zemel MB. The role of dairy foods in weight management. Journal of the American College of Nutrition 24(6 Suppl) (Dec 2005): 537S–46S. Review.

Zemel MB, Miller SL. Dietary calcium and dairy modulation of adiposity and obesity risk. Nutrition Reviews 62(4) (Apr 2004): 125–31.

Zemel MB, Richards J, Mathis S, Milstead A, Gebhardt L, Silva E. Dairy augmentation of total and central fat loss in obese subjects. International Journal of Obesity Related Metabolic Disorders 29(4) (Apr 2005): 391–7.

CHAPTER 7
Exercise: Why Smart Is Better than Long

Andersen RE. Exercise, an active lifestyle, and obesity. The Physician and Sportsmedicine 7(10) (1999). Available at http://www.physsportsmed.com/issues/1999/10-01-99/andersen.htm

Andersen RE, Blair SN, Cheskin LJ, et al. Encouraging patients to become more physically active: The physician's role. Annals of Internal Medicine 127(5) (1997): 395–400.

Andersen RE, Crespo CJ, Bartlett SJ, et al. Relationship of physical activity and television watching with body weight and level of fatness among children: Results from the Third National Health and Nutrition Examination Survey. Journal of the American Medical Association 279(12) (1998): 938–42.

Armstrong K, Edwards H. The effectiveness of a pram-walking exercise programme in reducing depressive symptomatology for postnatal women. International Journal of Nursing Practice 10(4) (Aug 2004): 177–94.

Bahr R, Sejersted OM. Effect of intensity of exercise on excess post-exercise oxygen consumption. Metabolism 40(8) (1991): 836–41.

Bahr R, Ingnes I, Vaage O, Sejersted OM, Newsholme EA. Effect of duration of exercise on excess post-exercise oxygen consumption. Journal of Applied Physiology 62(2) (1987): 485–90.

Ballor DL, Poehlman ET. A meta-analysis of the effects of exercise and/or dietary restriction on resting metabolic rate. European Journal of Applied Physiology 71(6) (1995): 535–42.

Borsheim E, Bahr R. Effect of exercise intensity, duration and mode on post-exercise oxygen consumption. Sports Medicine 33(14) (2003): 1037–60.

Braun WA, Hawthorne WE, Markofski MM. Acute EPOC response in women to circuit training and treadmill exercise of matched oxygen consumption. European Journal of Applied Physiology (Jun 8, 2005).

References

Chad KE, Wenger HA. The effect of exercise duration on the exercise and post-exercise oxygen consumption. Canadian Journal of Sport Science 13(4): 204–7.

Cordain L, Gotshall RW, Eaton SB. Evolutionary aspects of exercise. Nutrition and Fitness: Evolutionary Aspects. Children's Health. Programs and Policies. World Review of Nutrition and Dietetics. Basel, Karger. 81 (1997): 49–60.

Cordain L, Gotshall RW, Eaton SB, Eaton SB III. Physical activity, energy expenditure and fitness: An evolutionary perspective. International Journal of Sports Medicine 19 (1998): 328–35.

Crommett AD, Kinzey SJ. Excess postexercise oxygen consumption following acute aerobic and resistance exercise in women who are lean or obese. Journal of Strength and Conditioning Research 18(3) (Aug 2004): 410–15.

Cummings DE and Merriam GR. Growth hormone therapy in adults. Annual Review of Medicine 54 (2003): 513–33.

Drummond MJ, Vehrs PR, Schaalje GB, Parcell AC. Aerobic and resistance exercise sequence affects excess postexercise oxygen consumption. Journal of Strength and Conditioning Research 19(2) (May 2005): 332–7.

Elliot DL, Goldberg L, Kuehl KS. Effect of resistance training on excess postexercise oxygen consumption. Journal of Strength and Conditioning Research 6(2) (1992): 77–81.

Frey GC, Byrnes WC, Mazzeo RS. Factors influencing excess post-exercise oxygen consumption in trained and untrained women. Metabolism 42(7) (1993): 822–8.

Gilette CA, Bullough RC, Melby C. Post-exercise energy expenditure in response to acute aerobic or resistive exercise. International Journal of Sports Nutrition 4 (1994): 347–60.

Goto K, Ishii N, Kizuka T, Takamatzu K. The impact of metabolic stress on hormonal responses and muscular adaptations. Medicine and Science in Sports and Exercise 37(6) (2005): 955–63.

Godfrey RJ, Madgwick Z, Whyte GP. The exercise-induced growth hormone response in athletes. Sports Medicine 33(8) (2003): 599–613.

Gore CJ, Withers RT. The effect of exercise intensity and duration on the oxygen deficit and excess post-exercise oxygen consumption. European Journal of Applied Physiology and Occupational Physiology 60(3) (1990): 169–74.

Haltom RW, Kraemer RR, Sloan RA, Hebert EP, Frank K, Tryniecki JL. Circuit weight training and its effects on excess postexercise oxygen consumption. Medicine and Science in Sports and Exercise 31(11) (Nov 1999): 1613–18.

Holloszy JO, Kohrt WM, Hansen PA. The regulation of carbohydrate and fat metabolism during and after exercise. Frontiers in Bioscience 3 (Sep 15, 1998): D1011–27.

Holloway L, Butterfield G, Hintz RL, et al. Effect of recombinant human growth hormone on metabolic indices, body composition, and bone turnover in healthy elderly women. Journal of Clinical Endocrinology and Metabolism 79 (1994): 470–79.

Kaminsky LA, Whaley MH. Effect of interval type exercise on excess post-exercise oxygen consumption (EPOC) in obese and normal-weight women. Medicine in Exercise, Nutrition and Health 2 (1993): 106–11.

Laforgia J, Withers RT, Shipp NJ, Gore CJ. Comparison of exercise expenditure elevations after submaximal and supramaximal running. Journal of Applied Physiology 82(2) (1997): 661–6.

Lee CD, Blair SN, Jackson AS. Cardiorespiratory fitness, body composition, and all-cause and cardiovascular disease mortality in men. American Journal of Clinical Nutrition 69(3) (1999): 373–80.

Maehlum S, Grandmontagne M, Newsholme EA, Sejersted OM. Magnitude and duration of excess post exercise oxygen consumption in healthy young subjects. Metabolism 35(5) (1986): 425–9.

Marcus R, Hoffman AR. Growth hormone as therapy for older men and women. Annual Review of Pharmacology and Toxicology 38 (1998): 45–61.

Marzke MW, Longhill JM, Rasmussen SA. Gluteus maximus muscle function and the origin of hominid bipedality. American Journal of Physical Anthropology 77(4) (Dec 1988): 519–28.

Murphy E, Swartzkopf R. Effects of standard set and circuit weight training on excess post-exercise oxygen consumption. Journal of Applied Sport Science Research 6(2) (1992): 88–91.

Paluska SA, Schwenk TL. Physical activity and mental health: Current concepts. Sports Medicine 29(3) (Mar 2000): 167–80.

Papadakis MA, Grady D, Black D, et al. Growth hormone replacement in healthy older men improves body composition but not functional ability. Annals of Internal Medicine 124 (1996): 708–16.

Phelian JF, Reinke E, Harris MA, Melby CL. Post-exercise energy expenditure and substrate oxidation in young women resulting from exercise bouts of different intensity. Journal of the American College of Nutrition 16(2) (1997): 140–46.

Pollock ML, Franklin BA, Balady GJ, et al. Resistance exercise in individuals with and without cardiovascular disease: benefits, rationale, safety, and prescription: An advisory from the committee on exercise, rehabilitation, and prevention, Council on Clinical Cardiology, American Heart Association. Circulation 101(7) (2000): 828–33.

Pollock ML, Gaesser GA, Butcher JD, et al. The recommended quantity and quality of exercise for developing and maintaining cardiorespiratory and muscular fitness, and flexibility in healthy adults. Medicine and Science in Sports and Exercise 30(6) (1998): 975–91.

Pritzlaff CJ, Wideman L, Weltman JY, Abbott RD, Gutgesell ME, Hartman ML, Veldhuis JD, Weltman A. Impact of acute exercise intensity on pulsatile growth hormone release in men. Journal of Applied Physiology 87(2) (Aug 1999): 498–504.

Pritzlaff-Roy CJ, Widemen L, Weltman JY, Abbott R, Gutgesell M, Hartman ML, Veldhuis JD, Weltman A. Gender governs the relationship between exercise intensity and growth hormone release in young adults. Journal of Applied Physiology 92(5) (May 2002): 2053–60.

Quinn TJ, Vroman NB, Kertzer R. Post-exercise oxygen consumption in trained females: effect of exercise duration. Medicine and Science in Sports and Exercise 26(7) (1994): 908–13.

Romijn JA, Coyle EF, Sidossis LS, Zhang XJ, Wolfe RR. Relationship between fatty acid delivery and fatty acid oxidation during strenuous exercise. Journal of Applied Physiology 79(6) (Dec 1995): 1939–45.

Rudman D, Feller AG, Nagraj HS, et al. Effects of human growth hormone in men over 60 years old. New England Journal of Medicine 323 (1990): 1–6.

Schuenke MD, Mikat RP, McBride JM. Effect of an acute period of resistance exercise on excess post-exercise oxygen consumption: implications for body mass management. European Journal of Applied Physiology 86(5) (Mar 2002): 411–17.

Sedlock DA. Post-exercise energy expenditure after cycle ergometer and treadmill exercise. Journal of Applied Sport Science Research 6(1) (1992): 19–23.

Sedlock DA, Fissinger JA, Melby CL. Effect of exercise intensity and duration on post-exercise energy expenditure. Medicine and Science in Sports and Exercise 21(6) (1989): 662–6.

Smith J, McNaughton L. The effects of intensity of exercise on excess post-exercise oxygen consumption and energy expenditure in moderately trained men and women. European Journal of Applied Physiology 67 (1993): 420–25.

Stern JT Jr. Anatomical and functional specializations of the human gluteus maximus. American Journal of Physical Anthropology 36(3) (May 1972): 315–39.

Takala J, Ruokonen E, Webster NR, et al. Increased mortality associated with growth hormone treatment in critically ill adults. New England Journal of Medicine 341 (1999): 785–92.

Thornton MK, Potteiger JA. Effects of resistance exercise bouts of different intensities but equal work on EPOC. Medicine and Science in Sports and Exercise 34(4) (2002): 715–22.

US Department of Health and Human Services: Physical Activity and Health: A Report of the Surgeon General, Atlanta, DHHS, Centers for Disease Control and Prevention, National Center for Chronic Disease Prevention and Health Promotion (1996).

Vance ML, Mauras N. Drug therapy: Growth hormone therapy in adults and children. New England Journal of Medicine 341 (1999): 1206–16.

Withers RT, Gore CJ, Mackay MH, Berry MN. Some aspects of metabolism following a 35 km road run. European Journal of Applied Physiology and Occupational Physiology 63(6) (1991): 436–43.

You T, Nicklas BJ. Inflammation and the metabolic syndrome: Role of adipose tissue and modulation by exercise. Medicine and Science in Sports and Exercise 36(5) Suppl (May 2004): S1.

CHAPTER 8
The Ten Years Thinner Diet

Albert CM, Gaziano JM, Willett WC, Manson JE. Nut consumption and decreased risk of sudden cardiac death in the Physicians' Health Study. Archives of Internal Medicine 162(12) (Jun 24, 2002): 1382–7.

Cabrera C, Artacho R, Giménez R. Beneficial effects of green tea—A review. Journal of the American College of Nutrition 25(2) (2006): 79–99.

Chan J, Knutsen SF, Blix GG, Lee JW, Fraser GE. Water, other fluids, and fatal coronary heart disease: The Adventist Health Study. American Journal of Epidemiology 155 (2002): 827–33.

Cordain L. The nutritional characteristics of a contemporary diet based upon Paleolithic food groups. Journal of the American Neutraceutical Association 5 (2002): 15–24.

Curb JD, Wergowske G, Dobbs JC, Abbott RD, Huang B. Serum lipid effects of a high-monounsaturated fat diet based on macadamia nuts. Archives of Internal Medicine 160(8) (Apr 24, 2000): 1154–8.

Dean BB, Borenstein JE, Henning JM, Knight K, Merz CN. Can change in high-density lipoprotein cholesterol levels reduce cardiovascular risk? American Heart Journal 147(6) (Jun 2004): 966–76.

Fraser GE, Sabate J, Beeson WL, Strahan TM. A possible protective effect of nut consumption on risk of coronary heart disease. The Adventist Health Study. Archives of Internal Medicine 152(7) (Jul 1992): 1416–24.

Griel AE, Eissenstat B, Juturu V, Hsieh G, Kris-Etherton PM. Improved diet quality with peanut consumption. Journal of the American College of Nutrition 23(6) (2004): 660–68.

References

Hirano-Ohmori R, Rie Takahashi MS, Momiyama Y, Taniguchi H, Yonemura A, Tamai S, Umegaki K, Nakamura H, Kondo K, Ohsuzu F. Green tea consumption and serum malondialdehyde-modified LDL concentrations in healthy subjects. Journal of the American College of Nutrition 24(5) (2005): 342–6.

Johnston CS. Strategies for healthy weight loss: From vitamin C to the glycemic response. Journal of the American College of Nutrition 24(3) (Jun 2005): 158–65.

Klevay LM. Copper in nuts may lower heart disease risk. Archives of Internal Medicine 153(3) (Feb 8, 1993): 401–2.

Kritchevsky SB. A review of scientific research and recommendations regarding eggs. Journal of the American College of Nutrition 23(90006) (2004): 596S–600S.

Maniscalco BS, Taylor KA. Calcification in coronary artery disease can be reversed by EDTA-tetracycline long-term chemotherapy. Pathophysiology 11(2) (Oct 2004): 95–101. PMID: 15364120.

Olsson ME, Gustavsson KE, Andersson S, Nilsson A, Duan RD. Inhibition of cancer cell proliferation in vitro by fruit and berry extracts and correlations with antioxidant levels. Journal of Agricultural and Food Chemistry 52(24) (Dec 1, 2004): 7264–71.

Ródenas S, Rodríguez-Gil S, Merinero MC, Sánchez-Muniz FJ. Dietary exchange of an olive oil and sunflower oil blend for extra virgin olive oil decreases the estimate cardiovascular risk and LDL and apolipoprotein AII concentrations in postmenopausal women. Journal of the American College of Nutrition 24(5) (2005): 361–9.

Sabate J, Cordero-Macintyre Z, Siapco G, Torabian S, Haddad E. Does regular walnut consumption lead to weight gain? British Journal of Nutrition 94(5) (Nov 2005): 859–64.

Simopoulos AP, Salem N. Egg yolk as source of long-chain polyunsaturated fatty acids in infant feeding. American Journal of Clinical Nutrition 55(2) (Feb 1992): 411–14.

Sumpio BE, Cordova AC, Berke-Schlessel DW, Qin F, Chen QH. Green tea, the "Asian paradox," and cardiovascular disease. Journal of the American College of Surgeons 202(5) (May 2006): 813–25.

Tiwary CM, Ward JA, Jackson BA. Effect of pectin on satiety in healthy US Army adults. Journal of the American College of Nutrition 16(5) (Oct 1997): 423–8.

Vander Wal JS, Marth JM, Khosla P, Jen KLC, Dhurandhar NV. Short-term effect of eggs on satiety in overweight and obese subjects. Journal of the American College of Nutrition 24(6) (2005): 510–15.

Wu WH, Liu LY, Chung CJ, Jou HJ, Wang TA. Estrogenic effect of yam ingestion in healthy postmenopausal women. Journal of the American College of Nutrition 24(4) (2005): 235–43.

CHAPTER 9
The Ten Years Thinner Workout

Crust L. Carry-over effects of music in an isometric muscular endurance task. Perceptual and Motor Skills 98(3 Pt 1) (Jun 2004): 985–91.

CHAPTER 10
Forever Young

Greenfield JR, Samaras K, Jenkins AB, Kelly PJ, Spector TD, Campbell LV. Moderate alcohol consumption, dietary fat composition, and abdominal obesity in women: Evidence for gene-environment interaction. Journal of Clinical Endocrinology and Metabolism 88(11) (Nov 2003): 5381–6.

Laitinen J, Pietilainen K, Wadsworth M, Sovio U, Jarvelin MR. Predictors of abdominal obesity among 31-y-old men and women born in Northern Finland in 1966. European Journal of Clinical Nutrition 58(1) (Jan 2004): 180–90.

Leonard NH, Beauvais LL, Scholl RW. Work motivation: The incorporation of self based processes. Human Relations 52 (1999): 969–98.

Mukamal KJ, Chiuve SE, Rimm EB. Alcohol consumption and risk for coronary heart disease in men with healthy lifestyles. Archives of Internal Medicine 166(19) (Oct 23, 2006): 2145–50.

Suter PM. Is alcohol consumption a risk factor for weight gain and obesity? CRC Critical Reviews in Clinical Laboratory Sciences 42(3) (2005): 197–227.

———. Alcohol, lipid metabolism and body weight. Therapeutische Umschau 57(4) (Apr 2000): 205–11.

Theruvathu JA, Jaruga P, Nath RG, Dizdaroglu M, Brooks PJ. Polyamines stimulate the formation of mutagenic 1, N2-propanodeoxyguanosine adducts from acetaldehyde. Nucleic Acids Research 33(11) (Jun 21, 2005): 3513–20.

Twist C, Eston R. The effects of exercise-induced muscle damage on maximal intensity intermittent exercise performance. European Journal of Applied Physiology (May 11, 2005). Available at http://www.springerlink.com/content/u44ug2U248433401.